# HEALTHY DIVIDENDS

Investments in Nutrition, Movement,
and Healthy Habits that Pay Off

# HEALTHY DIVIDENDS

## Investments in Nutrition, Movement, and Healthy Habits that Pay Off

**TRICIA SILVERMAN, RD, MBA**

**Niche Pressworks**
Indianapolis

*Healthy Dividends: Investments in Nutrition, Movement, and Healthy Habits that Pay Off*

ISBN 978-1-946533-61-3 (ebook)
ISBN 978-1-946533-62-3 (paperback)
ISBN 978-1-946533-63-0 (hardback)

The stories in this book are about people I have worked with or met. Some of the names have been left out of the stories to protect the identities of those who have inspired and educated me through our work together.

For permission to reprint portions of this content or bulk purchases, contact Tricia Silverman at Tricia@TriciaSilverman.com

**Published by Niche Pressworks, Indianapolis, IN**

**NichePressworks.com**

Printed in the United States of America

# Dedication

For the Silverman boys, my husband and two sons, who gave me the gifts of time, patience, and understanding which helped me to complete this book.

# Acknowledgements

I want to thank Nicole of Niche Pressworks for helping to shape my ideas through the process of writing this book. I want to thank Kim of Niche Pressworks for helping me with the nuts and bolts of getting published, and the editors, Julie and Anna, who skillfully made my book more cohesive and enjoyable to read! A special thank you to Rebecca McCole who took the time to give me feedback on an early version of my book. Thank you to all the wonderful people with whom I have connected, named and unnamed in this book, who came to my seminars and shared stories and tips with me of what has helped them to achieve better health. Thanks to my wonderful mentors and role models, Lawrence Biscontini and Sara Kooperman, who have opened many doors for me. Thank you to my mom who kept health books and magazines around the house when I was growing up — which sparked my interest in nutrition. Thank you to my dad who, through his actions, showed that hard work pays off — the same way that investments in your health will pay off. And thank you to my husband, who served as both mom and dad while I traveled and wrote this book, and to my sons, who have taught me so much about life and love. And thanks to you, the reader, for picking up this book. I wrote this for you.

# Contents

Contents

# Preface

I was an overweight kid, and I didn't quite understand why. In hindsight, weekend overeating (more about that later in the book), my family showing love through food, and lunches lacking good nutrition all contributed to my horizontal growth. Splitting my pants and being called the Goodyear Blimp was not fun. Not wanting to become an obese adult, I found that the keys to winning at weight loss and wellness were eating more vegetables, moving my body, and other "investments" that I share in this book. This book will help you explore what others have found successful for them, so you can pick and choose which strategies you'll invest in for the long term. Your mix of investments will be different from your neighbor, family members, and co-workers. Your special mix of investments will give you many health returns and nutrition and longevity dividends.

The book will inspire you to look at wellness through different lenses and perspectives to help you eat more real food in reasonable amounts and less #Frankenfood (as in food that's been highly processed, conjuring up images of Frankenstein being created in a lab). It will also help you incorporate more movement, manage your weight, develop more healthful coping strategies, and get the most out of life.

Too much stress and not enough fun can lead to overeating, weight gain, and depression. Exploring the strategies in this book can help you tune into your food more, stop distracted eating, and set up an environment and habits that support health, and a long, vibrant life.

Thank you for investing in reading this book! I want you to get a return and dividends on this investment. Think about what the takeaways are for you, as you read each chapter. If you've attended one of my conference sessions, employee wellness seminars, or senior center presentations, this book will dive deeper and give you more than I can fit in my 60 or 90 minutes with you. If you've coached with me, this book can give you the support that's needed between calls. If we've never met, know that I've thoughtfully written this book to help inspire and guide you to a more healthful, nutritious life.

Let's get to work and earn some dividends!

—Tricia

# Introduction

Life is about making choices. Choosing to be healthy can sometimes feel complicated, but I'm here to tell you it doesn't have to be. A healthy choice can be as simple as deciding between a salad or a sandwich. The small choices you make every day add up to the habits and behaviors that can make you a happier, healthier person.

How do you do it? How do you make these choices? That's where I can help. I wrote this book to provide a resource and guide to healthy living: a place where you can find the answers. Note, I say healthy living because I believe that being healthy means taking care of every aspect of you. That means the whole package—nutrition, fitness, and weight management, and healthy habits. I view each of these elements as a way to invest in your health and future. Each investment supports the others and allows you to reap the dividends of health and wellness, which ultimately lead to longevity.

## Why Invest?

Three investments? That seems manageable, right? I would say unconditionally, yes, but I know from personal experience how hard it can be to sustain healthy commitments over time. That's another reason I've written this book and why I want you to keep the big picture in mind. Being healthy isn't a one-and-done deal. It's an investment in yourself with long-term dividends.

In each of the book's sections on Nutrition, Fitness and Weight Management, and Healthy Habits, I provide detailed strategies to help you understand the steps that will get you from where you are to where you want to be. I explain the investments you can make that will give you the dividends you want.

I've always been inspired by cultures where people have discovered the right mix of activity, food choices, and lifestyle. I like to call these longevity cultures. Some examples include Loma Linda, California, Mediterranean countries, Hunza, Pakistan, and Okinawa, Japan. Luckily, you don't have to live in these places to obtain the benefits of longevity. In fact, just a few small changes in your diet, activity, and lifestyle can go a long way. For more detailed information about some of these cultures, go to appendix A.

## Longevity

Picture yourself in your golden years. Do you want to be living on your own, perhaps doing yoga, dancing, traveling, and enjoying life to the fullest? Through teaching about healthy aging for Northeastern University and presenting to and learning from active agers at senior centers, I have developed strategies that will help keep your dancing or golf shoes on until your 90s and beyond.

A great example of living life to the fullest through investing in healthy habits is Caster Salemi. He's 97 years young and still driving, socializing, and enjoying an active, fun life. Caster appears to be in his early 80s. When I first met him, I was blown away to discover he was in his 90s! He is mentally sharp with a positive attitude, great memory, and a sense of humor. You can view impromptu interviews with him on my website and Facebook page.

Caster is a living example of how good health can impact your life. He lives the Mediterranean lifestyle, still cooks for his daughter, drives, and goes to yoga. In between all of those activities, he attends social events at different senior centers. Adapting healthful habits now can help you to live a long, fruitful life into your 90s, just like Caster!

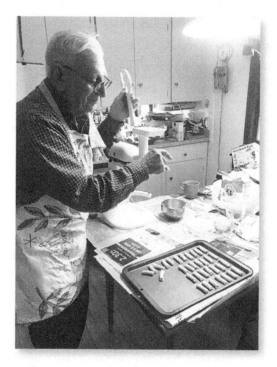

*Caster Salemi, baking in his kitchen at 96 years old.*

**Other Long-Term Dividends Include:**

**Less Money Spent on Medication** – Why go on medication to solve health issues when you may not have to? The more medications you are on, the more side effects and drug interactions you must worry about. Especially as you get older, the cost of medications can take a large chunk of your income. By eating well and exercising, you improve your health and decrease the risk of health-related problems.

## Goodbye Medication, High Blood Pressure, High Cholesterol, and Pain! Hello, New Life!

Fourteen years ago, Elizabeth Petruccione was literally killing herself with food after a tumultuous six-month period where she lost her son, her sister, and her job. She said she was going to "eat until I die." As time went by, Elizabeth's health deteriorated, and her weight hit an all-time high of 248 pounds. While carrying around extra weight, Elizabeth was seeing a chiropractor and physical therapist regularly for severe rheumatoid arthritis and pain in her lower back. She also had shoulder pain from stooping over, and kept breaking her toes. She was paying over $1,000 a year in copays for pain medication and other medications.

Through her own strategies, she lost 68 pounds in eight months. She then joined a national weight loss program, attended its meetings, and lost 30 additional pounds in 27 months. Attending the meetings was a key success factor for her. She went on to lead weight loss meetings for the same company. She then opened her own business, helping inspire people to lose weight.

Elizabeth is now a svelte 158 pounds and has seen tremendous financial savings since she no longer has so many copays for medication. Losing weight helped rid pain and arthritis in her back, as well as her sleep apnea, high blood pressure, cholesterol, and acid reflux. And what about physical therapy or trips to the chiropractor? Now she never has to go! She attributes the reduction of her pain to losing weight, eating nutritious food, and exercising. She trains with weights and has strengthened her back to make it stronger.

Elizabeth possesses a unique wisdom about weight loss. She has a gravitational pull — perhaps she is the pied piper (or pipess) of weight loss. She shares her wise thoughts about weight loss and maintenance — which I've coined as dietisms. You'll read about these later in the book.

**Elizabeth Before  Elizabeth After**

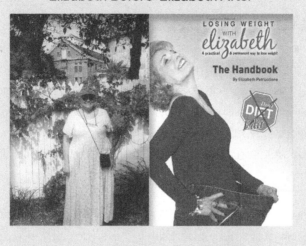

**Lower Cholesterol, Blood Pressure, Blood Sugars** – Are you looking for a pill to solve your health issues? Too many people look for the quick fix and end up quickly disappointed. Pills often don't solve the root causes of your health issues. If you take cholesterol medication but continue to eat large "boot-long" meat-filled sub sandwiches, you're not getting to the root cause. Good habits are natural remedies that treat the source of your illness.

**More Mobility and Independence** – Wouldn't it feel nice to be able to drive a new car around when you're in your 90s? When I gave my longevity seminar, *Longevity Gifts of Abkhazia, Vilcabamba,* *and Hunza,* at the Sterling Senior Center in Massachusetts, I shared the healthy habits and food preferences of these cultures. Little did I know that there was a person in the audience who personified our discussion. I spoke about how the elders in these cultures keep moving and doing what they can. They do things like tend animals, work the land, garden, walk in nature, and stay active.

**Be Like Ken!** At the end of the seminar at Sterling Senior Center, a couple of active agers came up to chat with me. One was Ken Day, a retired duck farmer in his 90s at the time, who was living the life! The person at his side was Ken's hot, younger girlfriend — in her 80s! Ken shared that vegetables are part of what he eats every day, and he pulled his preferred snack of nuts out of his pocket. Ken was active on social media and was driving a new car.

Fast forward to my recent call with Ken. He's now 102 and is still driving. He stays active by visiting the senior center every day where he shoots pool or does projects. Ken plays games such as Wii Bowling. He goes to church regularly and shared, "I'm a believer in the Lord." He goes to restaurants, loves to read, and for exercise, walks on the track or in the mall and lifts weights. "I do it a funny way," Ken said, referring to the fact that he does his weight-lifting while eating.

Ken shared that he never smoked or drank and that he likes to be around people. Ken has owned a computer since they first came out, and currently uses a laptop. He recommends going to bed and getting up at reasonable times and also putting thought into what you eat. He eats salmon twice a week and no red meat. He eats vegetables and fruit, and almost every day, he eats an applesauce that includes the apple peel.

Ken does not add salt, pepper, or sugar to his foods. He has decreased his portions as he has gotten older and has weighed the same for 25 years. Ken eats a healthy diet and also enjoys a one-cup portion of ice cream every other day. Planning for and enjoying small indulgences is a healthy and balanced way of enjoying life. You, too, can enjoy a long healthy life by learning from Ken's example.

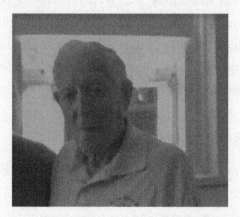

*Ken at the Sterling Senior Center in 2014*

**Feeling More in Control** – Have you ever felt like food was controlling you? With the *Healthy Dividends* strategies, you will feel more in control. We have too many food choices at supermarkets. Even some of the healthier supermarkets have become food carnivals. At one well-known healthy supermarket, they strategically installed a doughnut operation at the entrance of the store. Unhealthy visual stimuli can make it difficult to make good choices.

**Improved Productivity** – Your productivity at home and work can be dramatically improved when you replace habits that aren't serving you with healthy habits that are. Eating well and sleeping well help you concentrate and focus. Decreasing sugar intake can have an incredible impact on your daily productivity and energy.

**Increased Energy** – Are you fueling your day or your sleep? One of the best ways we can master our bodies and brains is to fuel ourselves when we are hungry, and need energy for brainwork and physical demands. Too many people make the mistake of not giving their bodies energy when they need it and end up overcompensating at their evening meal. This meal is often followed by sedentary behavior and sleep. By implementing smart nutrition timing, eating the right foods, and getting the movement and sleep your body needs, you will be rewarded with more energy.

## Keep It in Perspective

Through my work, I get to meet some amazing people — clients, seminar attendees, and coaches, to name a few. I learn a lot from these interactions, and one, in particular, comes to mind. I was speaking at the SCW Fitness Conference in Florida when I met Niko Provistalis, a personal trainer of Greek descent from Florida. As we discussed fitness, he made an interesting observation by noting that people in Greece are healthy and considered normal weight, even though they don't have the ripped and cut look that many strive for in the United States. That comment stuck with me.

I think many of us strive for a look that may be too hard to achieve, rather than a look that comes from realistic healthy eating and realistic healthy movement. Years ago, I read *Living Younger Longer* by the staff of Canyon Ranch Health Spa and Len Sherman. One of the ranch's philosophies, in particular, had an impact on me: "Your ideal weight is your weight after a period of time in which you 1) eat as well as you can reasonably eat, and 2) exercise as much as you can reasonably exercise."[1]

This makes so much sense to me, and I hope it gives comfort to you so that you can reach and attain what is reasonable for you. It helps to recognize that someone who enjoys bodybuilding is likely to have a different standard of what is reasonable than you or me, and that's okay. You just need to find what is reasonable for you.

In this book, you'll see how some more movement may be reasonable for you and improving and adapting some nutrition and well-being habits may also be reasonable. You'll find information and tools to help you set your course.

To help navigate the change, the book is organized into three categories: Nutrition, Fitness and Weight Management, and Healthy Habits. In each of these sections, the chapters provide detailed information as well as strategies and approaches to help you make healthy choices, so you can live a long, healthy, and energetic life. As you read the book, know that I am with you every step of the way. By investing in each of these areas, you'll find a wealth of happiness and health awaits.

Let's get started.

# INVESTMENT:
## NUTRITION

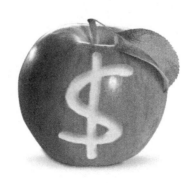

# CHAPTER 1

# NuTricia's Way of Eating!

## The Nuts and Bolts of the NuTricia's Way of Eating

There's some truth to the old saying that, "You are what you eat." The foods we eat, quite literally, provide the fuel our bodies use for all of our activities. How are you fueling your body? What types of foods do you eat? When I meet with new clients, I start by talking about the basics of nutrition. That means, we discuss what they frequently eat, and we make adjustments to move them toward optimal nutrition via the NuTricia's Way of Eating. Essentially, I help clients follow a balanced style of eating that provides the nutrients needed to thrive physically and mentally, which also pays dividends by helping them to live a long, flourishing life!

I've discovered that many people are losing long-term health benefits by following short-term, less than healthy diets. Those fad diets that say "No carbs" or "No fruit" may be robbing you of longevity, clear vibrant skin, and boundless health. In my many years as a nutritionist, I've witnessed a lot of unhealthy approaches to eating. I've visited homes where the pantry and refrigerator were completely empty. One woman ate all of her meals at donut shops, and her skin reflected this. She looked much older than her age, and her skin appeared dull and lifeless, as did her eyes. These are just some of the effects of poor eating habits.

In contrast, when giving a seminar at a senior center, I met an active ager who was a vegetarian. His skin was radiant, and his eyes sparkled. He was at least 30 years older than the woman I mentioned above who preferred donuts, yet his skin and eyes were more vibrant. The way you eat and how much you move shows through your eyes, skin, and attitude.

When you are healthfully nourishing your body, it shows in your health and movements. When you eat in extremes, your health can deteriorate. I worked with one client who primarily ate scones and grilled cheese for her meals, day in and day out. When she came to me, she wondered why the scale wouldn't budge. After tracking her meals, I was able to help her identify that her diet was very limited. Baked goods and cheesy grilled sandwiches pack a lot of calories into a seemingly small amount of food. It can be deceiving. I worked with her to add more variety into her diet: specifically vegetables and fruits, and healthy sources of protein, along with whole grains. When your plate is piled with vegetables, you get to eat more food for fewer calories. It's quite a beautiful thing!

## BONUS CONTENT!

Hope you are enjoying the book so far. To read the free Bonus Chapter, go to

**TriciaSilverman.com/book**

## NuTricia's Plate

In 2011, the USDA replaced its food pyramid with a new icon for healthy eating called MyPlate. It was designed to provide an easier way for people to understand and create balanced meals. The MyPlate icon shows an image of a place setting with a plate and glass. The plate is divided into food group targets (vegetables, protein, fruits, and grains). Shifting to a plate-based approach to nutrition encourages people to look at what's on their actual food plate. If your plate looks similar to the icon with lots of fruits and vegetables, then you're probably on the right track.

Since the USDA started its plate-based system, more specific and individualized ways to create the best healthy plate have become available. After working with hundreds of clients, I developed my own NuTricia's Plate, which reflects a balanced, success-driven approach to eating that allows you to live your best life.

Using the NuTricia's Plate strategy, half of your plate should be vegetables, one-fourth whole grains, and one-fourth protein. On the side, I suggest a serving of fruit and water (nature's beverage). In moderation, I suggest small amounts of fats, including nuts, seeds, nut butters, avocados, and organic oils (such as extra virgin olive oil and organic canola oil). Vegetables, fruits, whole grains, and beans should make up the bulk of the carbohydrates you are consuming.

# NuTricia's Plate

Three different fruits per day

Stay hydrated by drinking water (nature's beverage)

## Protein-Rich Foods.

Beans, Fish, Chicken, Turkey, Eggs, Nuts, Seeds, Limited Red Meat, Dairy (if tolerated)

## Carb-Rich Foods

Whole Grains (brown rice, millet, oatmeal, quinoa, whole wheat, etc.)

Starchy Vegetables (corn, peas, potatoes)

## Non-Starchy Vegetables

Salad Greens, Cooking Greens, Asparagus, Bok Choy, Broccoli, Carrots, Cabbage, Cauliflower, Celery, Cucumber, Eggplant, Mushrooms, Zucchini, etc. (At least 3 different vegetables per day)

Healthy Fats (in small amounts) such as Nuts, Seeds, Avocado, Extra Virgin Olive Oil, Organic Canola Oil, etc.

Supplements (as needed) such as Vitamin D, calcium, etc.

© 2019 Tricia Silverman

I've also incorporated into my plate, icons representing other aspects of a healthy life. A sunshine icon reminds you that sun (in moderation) is good for you and can help you produce Vitamin D. The person walking encourages you to keep moving during the day. Taking a walk after your meal can make your cells more responsive to the action of insulin, helping to control your blood sugar levels. A mindfulness and yoga icon reminds us that these can help you to create more body awareness and make better food choices. In the long term, practicing yoga may even have a positive effect on your hunger and fullness hormones. The dancing and music icons represent joy for life. We should have fun, sing, dance, and enjoy. Fun is an important part of life, and a good reminder that there is more to life than food or "dieting." Go out and have some fun!!

## Wellness Guidelines Work

Government-issued wellness guidelines offer helpful information based on what scientists currently know. The premise is that people can be healthy by following the U.S. Dietary and Physical Activity Guidelines. But, is that really true? One fitness writer, Daniel Green, decided to find out. He followed the U.S. Dietary and Physical Activity Guidelines for one year. During that time, he lost 34 pounds and over five inches off his waist. His health improved as well. His blood pressure, which had been high, returned to normal, and he went from prediabetes to normal blood sugar levels. Check out his inspiring story on Instagram at **www.Instagram.com/DanGreenWeighsIn/.**

# Food Groups

## Vegetables

At the absolute minimum, eat three different color vegetables every day. Ideally, you should eat between two and three cups of cooked vegetables and even more if you eat a lot of raw vegetables. Most people are not eating enough vegetables. Eating vegetables is one of the universal success factors for disease prevention, weight management, and longevity. Can you make this one of your investments?

## Fruits

For optimal health, you should eat between one and a half to two cups of fruit a day. This can be divided into half cup servings. A serving is roughly half cup or a small piece of fruit. To keep things easy, just remember to eat at least three different kinds of fruit per day. Fruit should be varied throughout the week as well.

Three servings of fruit per day can help strengthen your immune system, protect against cancer, and protect against macular degeneration. Dr. Allen Banik, an optometrist who visited the longevity culture Hunza in the 1950s (more about this culture in appendix A), found that the elder Hunzans had very healthy eyes.[2] No surprise because apricots were one of the popular fruits consumed in Hunza, and they contain carotenenoids — nutrients known to foster good eye health. Make sure to eat orange and yellow fruits and vegetables to get more of these nutritional gems.

Eating fruit can also help satisfy sweet cravings, which is a big help as you decrease (and eliminate) processed sweet foods from your diet. If you eat dried fruit, look for brands that do not have preservatives or unnecessary additives. Organic is a great bet! If you have a Trader Joe's near you, check out their delicious organic Turkish apricots. While dried fruit is healthy, it can be easy to eat too much, so portion it out or opt for fresh instead. Frozen fruit is helpful, especially for smoothies; however, try to eat mainly fresh fruit.

## Whole Grains

When it comes to grains, it's important to choose whole grains. They will help you to live longer, can contribute to a better mood, and protect you against heart disease and cancer. An easy way to know that you're eating the right kind of grains is to look for the word "whole" in the ingredient list, such as whole wheat, whole rye, and whole oats. If you see "enriched" on the ingredient list, run the other way!

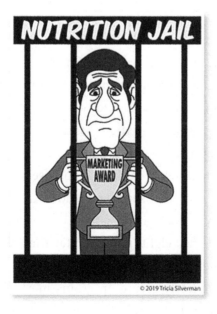

*The genius who came up with the word "enriched" for unhealthy white flour should win a "most misleading marketing" award and head straight to nutrition jail.*

Enriched flour means the bran and germ components (and most of the wonderful nutrients and fiber) were stripped away from the grain, and only some nutrients were added back. Companies strip away these elements to create a longer shelf life and a more pleasing texture for the processed foods that tend to tempt us most—cookies, crackers, pastry, cakes, bagels, rolls, white pasta, white rice—you get the idea.

Eat whole grains to get nutrients in their natural state, such as B vitamins, vitamin E, and iron. Here are some examples to shop for: old-fashioned or steel-cut oats, hulled (but not pearled) barley, brown rice, and breads, flours, or pastas that use the word "whole" in the ingredient list, such as whole wheat flour, whole wheat, whole rye, whole grain amaranth, whole grain spelt, whole grain corn meal, whole grain quinoa, etc. In Canada, when buying *whole wheat*, the label should also say *whole grain*, as food processors are allowed to remove some of the germ and bran and still call it *whole wheat*. However, they can't do this if the label says *whole grain*. Also, be wary of the word *multigrain*. This is a confusing term, and the product may or may not be whole grain. Multi- just means many, and it simply may mean many enriched grains. Read the ingredient list to be sure.

How much grain you should eat every day depends on the individual. US guidelines recommend four servings if you eat 1200 calories per day, and the servings gradually increase as calories increase to 10 servings for those eating 3200 calories per day. When you're looking to lose weight, going lighter than this may be helpful, especially as you get older.

However, completely giving up grains may affect your mood. A personal trainer friend of mine messaged me to tell me his girlfriend started practicing the Paleo (high protein/low carb) way of eating, and her mood had gone south! He asked for my advice. Can you guess what I told him? Add some carbs back. A serving of grain is typically a third cup serving of rice/pasta, one half cup cooked cereal, like oatmeal, or one slice of bread or three quarters cup of dry cereal. I have found myself cutting my portion sizes to help me keep my weight down, particularly as I age. So, if you are looking to lose weight, if a typical serving of cereal is three quarters cup, you may want to opt for a half cup.

## Protein

Consuming adequate protein is important for many reasons. Protein provides the amino acids which build muscles, gives structure to your cells, contributes to enzymes and hormones, helps transport and send messages within your body, repairs injuries, and keeps your immune system functioning. It can be used as an energy source if your diet is lacking carbohydrates and fats, and can be stored as fat if you eat more than you move.

Protein also helps you to feel fuller, so it is a good idea to have it be a part of your meals and snacks. The amount of protein to eat depends on your age and weight, as well as your weight loss and fitness goals.

### How Much Protein Do You Need?

It's a good idea to aim for at least 1 gram of protein per kilogram of your body weight. To get kilograms take your weight in pounds and divide by 2.2.

The RDA (Recommended Dietary Allowance) for protein is .8 grams per kilogram (or .36 grams per pound); however, this may be too low, especially if you're very active (which is the goal).

In general, use the following as a helpful guide for figuring out how many grams of protein to eat per day (Please note that protein grams are usually figured out based on body weight in kilograms. I have provided conversions to grams per pound, and rounded off in order to make the calculations easier):

- 1 gram of protein per kilogram of body weight (.45 grams per pound)

- If you do a lot of endurance activity, 1.2–1.4 g/kg (.54–.64 grams per pound) of body weight

- If you frequently lift weights and are looking to build muscle 1.4–2.0 g/kg (.64 –.91 grams per pound) body weight

**Example:**

Let's say you are a female weighing 150 pounds.

150 pounds/ 2.2 = 68.2 kilograms

Let's say you are looking to build muscle.

68.2 kg * 1.4 = 95.5 grams or 150 pounds * .64 = 96 grams

68.2 kg * 2.0 = 136.4 grams or 150 pounds * .91 = 136.5 grams

**You need roughly between 96 and 136 grams of protein per day to achieve your goals.**

For my detail-oriented friends, go with the grams per kilogram calculation! Everyone else, use the grams per pound and move on!

The following chart shows you the grams of protein in various foods:

**Sources of Protein, and Grams per Common Serving Sizes**

| Protein Sources | Grams of Protein in common serving sizes |
|---|---|
| Fish, shellfish, chicken, turkey, beef (3 oz.) | 21 |
| Beans, ½ cup cooked | 7 |
| Dairy products, 1 cup milk<br>Yogurt, 8 oz., nonfat plain<br>Yogurt, 8 oz., Greek, nonfat | 8<br>10<br>22 |
| Eggs, 1 | 6 |
| Grains, cooked ½–1/3 cup | 3 |
| Vegetables, non-starchy ½ cup cooked<br>Starchy (e.g., corn, peas) ½ cup cooked | 2<br>3 |
| Soy products, Soy milk (8 oz.)<br>Tofu (3 oz.) | 7<br>7 |

*Sources of protein and grams of protein in common serving sizes*

Two sources of protein that have outstanding health benefits are fish and beans. Aim for at least two fish meals per week (more about fish in the "Feed Your Brain" section of chapter 7). Beans are a food of longevity, packed with micronutrients and fiber. They help decrease cholesterol levels and constipation. The Paleo way of eating discourages eating beans. I disagree with this approach. Beans are a staple in many areas of longevity.

Red meat includes pork, beef, and lamb. No, pork truly is not "the other white meat," as the old saying goes. Again, someone deserves a marketing award while being locked up in Nutrition Jail. These meats are associated with cancer, heart disease, and earlier mortality.

Processed red meats, like bacon and cold cuts, are even worse than unprocessed. It's a good idea to limit red meat in your diet. One of the best things you can do for your health is to replace meat with protein-rich, plant-based options. Even eating non-meat meals a few times a week can have a big impact on your health. I like to make black beans with brown rice and spinach. I mix in a small amount peanut or almond butter thinned out with some water, and a sprinkle of garlic, ginger, and crushed red pepper—a quick and tasty Thai-inspired meal.

## Healthy Fats

Fat is essential. It's not the 1980s anymore when you might have gone fat-free. The fat consumed in food is a source of energy, helps you absorb vitamins A, D, E, and K, and helps make you full. It also provides essential fatty acids, such as omega-3 fats, that your body needs but can't make on its own.

Dietary fats in food are organized into three categories—polyunsaturated, monounsaturated, and saturated fatty acids. Fats are classified based on their chemical structures. Although oils such as olive oil contain elements of all three categories, oils are often referred to by the type of fat that they contain most. For example, olive oil is often referred to as a monounsaturated fat, since most of the fatty acids in olive oil are monounsaturated, but it also contains some saturated and polyunsaturated fatty acids. Most oils primarily contain unsaturated fatty acids, though they often have small amounts of saturated fatty acids (exceptions are coconut oil, palm kernel and palm oil, which contain predominately saturated fatty acids, a reason to consume them only in small amounts).

You've probably heard these words, but they didn't quite make sense. Let's take a closer look at fats to figure out which ones to eat and which ones to avoid.

## Desirable Fats – Monounsaturated and Polyunsaturated

Monounsaturated and some polyunsaturated fats are associated with living longer![3] A subclass of polyunsaturated fats that particularly support optimal health are the omega-3 fats. Omega-3 fats are anti-inflammatory, are important structural components of brain cells, and help protect against heart disease, Alzheimer's, and other conditions related to inflammation. These fats may also help support a better mood.

Omega-3 fats are found in high amounts in fatty fish such as salmon, herring, trout, bluefish, anchovies, and sardines. Eating eight ounces of fish over the course of the week is a great goal. Plant-based sources of omega-3 fats are found in walnuts, pumpkin seeds, chia seeds, hemp seeds, organic canola oil, and soy foods.

## Choose these Foods to Get More Unsaturated Fats in Your Diet:

- **Oils:** Extra virgin olive oil is the oil that has the most scientific evidence available supporting its health benefits. When choosing oils, look for expeller (mechanically) pressed and/or organic oils. Oils that are not expeller pressed may be extracted using harsh chemicals. Besides olive oil, other oils high in monounsaturated fats include canola, peanut, sunflower, and safflower oils.
- **Avocados, Nuts and Seeds, Nut and Seed Butters, and Olives**
- **Fatty Fish:** salmon, herring, trout, bluefish, anchovies, sardines

## Undesirable Fats – Saturated Fats

These are the bad fats associated with higher cholesterol levels. Animal foods are abundant in saturated fats, including meat, cheese, and dairy foods. Most research concurs that saturated fat should be limited to less than 10 percent of the calories you consume. See the table on the next page for daily limits (in grams) of saturated fat, depending on how many calories you are eating.

Most of the evidence-based research still indicates that choosing lower-fat dairy products is a wise choice, since whole and two-percent milk and most cheeses contain a significant amount of saturated fat. This means it's also a good idea to limit butter usage since it is high in saturated fat. Think about where you use butter or margarine, and think about whether you can use something healthier instead. For instance, if you eat butter on toast, could you make avocado toast or spread almond butter on your toast?

When purchasing lower fat dairy products, be careful to read the ingredient list. Sometimes unnecessary fillers, such as starches, gums, and sweeteners are added when the fat is reduced. In general, choose products that have a short ingredient list. Compare labels. If you enjoy the full-fat versions of dairy, keep your portions small and lower the rest of the day's intake of saturated fat rich foods. Limit use of high saturated fat oils, such as coconut oil, palm oil, and palm kernel oil.

- **Trans Fats:** These occur naturally in some animal foods and are also an additive in foods. This additive starts as an oil and is then chemically manipulated to make it more solid. It has been associated with heart disease and should be avoided. Even though labels may say 0 trans fats, there has been a loophole that allows companies to claim 0 trans fats if there are less than .5 grams per serving. Therefore, it's important to look beyond the numbers on the food label and take a closer look at the ingredient list. Look for the words "partially hydrogenated" in the ingredient label and run away as fast as you can! Processed foods like baked goods and crackers may have trans fats. Food manufacturers are supposed to stop using trans fats in manufacturing by January 2021.

## How Much Fat Should You Eat?

The Institute of Medicine says that the acceptable range of fat intake is between 20 to 35 percent of someone's diet. This range includes a variety of diets. Vegans may be on the low end of fat intake, while those following the Mediterranean Diet may be at the higher end. The popular Keto diet does not stay in this range, which is one of the reasons I don't recommend it. As mentioned previously, saturated fat should be limited to less than 10 percent of total calories.

The table below shows the fat grams recommended based on the calories consumed.

| Calories Per Day | Fat Grams Per Day (20–35% of total calories) | Saturated Fat Grams Per Day (less than 10% of total calories) |
|---|---|---|
| 1,400 | Between 31g and 54 g | Less than 16 g |
| 1,600 | Between 36 g and 62 g | Less than 18 g |
| 1,800 | Between 40 g and 70 g | Less than 20 g |
| 2,000 | Between 44 g and 78 g | Less than 22 g |
| 2,200 | Between 49 g and 86 g | Less than 24 g |
| 2,400 | Between 53 g and 93 g | Less than 27 g |

Let's say you enjoy avocados, nuts, seeds, and extra virgin olive oil as your main sources of fat. Let's look at a few examples of how much fat is in some healthy fat-rich food items:

| Serving Size | Food | Total Fat (grams) | Saturated Fat (grams) |
|---|---|---|---|
| ⅓ medium | Avocado | 7 | 1 |
| 1 oz. or ¼ cup | Almonds | 14 | 1 |
| 1 teaspoon | Extra virgin olive oil | 5 | .5 |
| 4 oz. | Wild salmon | 9 | 1.5 |
| Total: | | 35 | 4 |

If you were to eat all of the above, your total fat grams consumed would be 35 grams, and total saturated fat would be 4 grams. If you are eating a diet of 1,400 calories, you are meeting the guidelines.

## Is Coconut Oil Okay to Eat?

One of the oils that has gained a lot of popularity recently is coconut oil. This is one of the most saturated oils. You can still use it, just watch your portions. A typical coconut oil label will say that one tablespoon has 120 calories and 14 grams of total fat; 12 grams of the fat is saturated fat. If you are following a 1,600 calorie diet, the recommended limit on saturated fat grams **is less than 18 grams**. The 12 grams in the coconut oil is close to this limit, so the rest of the day's food should be low in saturated fat.

## Fluid Guidelines

Are you drinking enough water? Drinking more water is a relatively easy change you can make that pays enormous dividends. Drinking more water is an investment that has supported weight loss for many of my clients. One way to do this is to set water cues to remind you to drink more. For example, leave a cup in the bathroom so every time you go, you then drink water to replenish. Keeping a cup or water bottle on your desk or kitchen counter can also help you drink more water.

Proper hydration is important to prevent dehydration and constipation and helps you move and think clearly.[4] It also helps the appearance and integrity of your skin. Water is essential for survival and is involved in metabolism, transport of oxygen, nutrients, and waste products in your body, as well as fluid balance.[5] The sensation of thirst often diminishes with age, so relying on thirst as an indicator to replenish fluids may not be accurate.

## How Much?

There is no consensus on how to estimate fluid needs for adults. The typical eight glasses of water a day is a helpful goal. Another way to figure out if you're getting enough is to look at your pee and notice its color and odor. If it is pale to light yellow, you are good. If it gets darker than this, then you probably need to drink more water. If your urine has a strong odor that could indicate you need more water (or you ate some asparagus!).

Water is nature's beverage, and most of your fluid should come from it. When you are hungry and trying to lose weight, try drinking some water first. You might have just been thirsty without realizing it. In the valuable classic book *Food & Mood* by Elizabeth Somer,

Registered Dietitian, she says that a desire for sweets in the evening may just be an indication that your body needs more fluid.[6] One to two glasses of cold water may decrease an ice cream craving.

## Nutrition Staircase

I developed the NuTricia's Healthy Eating Staircase to show how we are all at different steps on the nutrition staircase. And, the staircase never ends … we just keep wanting to move up. Where are you on the staircase? Would you like to incorporate some of the nutrition tips talked about above into your nutrition staircase?

### From Milkshake Connoisseur to Buff MD

When I first met William Borde-Perry, or Dr. Will, I noticed his sculpted body was strikingly similar to LL Cool J's. Along with the muscles, he was wearing cool running shoes that looked like feet, the kind that have an individual spot for each toe. I naturally assumed he was a fitness instructor. Since I had heard mixed reviews about those types of shoes and had never seen anyone actually wearing them, I asked him about the shoes. I found out that Will was an ER doctor and had an uplifting and motivating success story behind those shoes and muscles … and, yes, he gives a thumbs up to the shoes!

Before medical school, Dr. Will weighed in the low 200 pound range before topping out at around 230 pounds when he graduated from his residency. Post-residency, with his work schedule of rotating emergency room shifts throughout the day

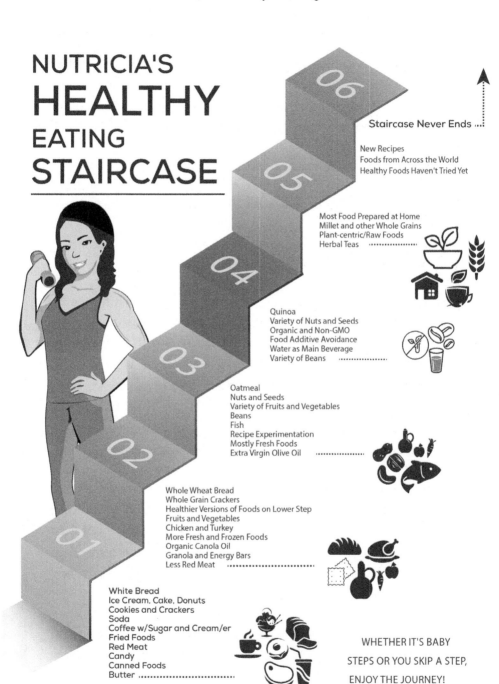

# NUTRICIA'S
# HEALTHY
# EATING
# STAIRCASE

**06**

Staircase Never Ends ....

New Recipes
Foods from Across the World
Healthy Foods Haven't Tried Yet

**05**

Most Food Prepared at Home
Millet and other Whole Grains
Plant-centric/Raw Foods
Herbal Teas ....................

**04**

Quinoa
Variety of Nuts and Seeds
Organic and Non-GMO
Food Additive Avoidance
Water as Main Beverage
Variety of Beans ....................

**03**

Oatmeal
Nuts and Seeds
Variety of Fruits and Vegetables
Beans
Fish
Recipe Experimentation
Mostly Fresh Foods
Extra Virgin Olive Oil ....................

**02**

Whole Wheat Bread
Whole Grain Crackers
Healthier Versions of Foods on Lower Step
Fruits and Vegetables
Chicken and Turkey
More Fresh and Frozen Foods
Organic Canola Oil
Granola and Energy Bars
Less Red Meat ..............................

**01**

White Bread
Ice Cream, Cake, Donuts
Cookies and Crackers
Soda
Coffee w/Sugar and Cream/er
Fried Foods
Red Meat
Candy
Canned Foods
Butter ..............................

WHETHER IT'S BABY
STEPS OR YOU SKIP A STEP,
ENJOY THE JOURNEY!

and night, it was easiest for him to go to fast food joints to refuel between shifts. He particularly enjoyed milkshakes and boasts that he could give you an amazing review and comparison of each milkshake from all of the fast food venues.

## Milk (and Belly) Shakes No More

A turning point for Dr. Will was in August 2009 when he weighed around 265. He had a spare tire and 42-inch waist, His clothes didn't fit, and his daughter punched his belly while letting everyone know that "Daddy has a fat belly."

Sitting in his living room, an infomercial for Shaun T.'s Insanity 60-day DVD fitness program intrigued him. "It was the hardest workout on TV. I've never seen anything like it. People were practically passing out and falling down." This was all really fascinating to him. "I was embarrassed to buy it since I normally don't buy anything off the TV." But he did it. He bought the program, survived the Insanity challenge, and then moved on to Tony Horton's popular 90-day P90X DVD workout.

In January 2010, with his fitness program well underway, Dr. Will was ready for the next step—changing his diet. With the help of a nutritionist and various self-help and fitness books, he modified what he ate. The internet was also very helpful. Once he got started, he realized, "No one has any excuse. Calorie and nutrition info are readily available."

Dr. Will eats three meals and two snacks a day. His protein sources are mainly chicken and fish since beef doesn't seem to digest as well for him. He eats lots of vegetables, not too much bread, and stays away from fried foods. As for fruit, Dr. Will says, "I use it to kill my craving for candy, while I'm also getting valuable antioxidants, vitamins, and minerals." He reads labels, tracks what he eats, and sets daily protein goals to guide his food choices. Dr. Will shares that "Protein makes you full faster." He also uses the Daily Burn app on his phone to look at labels.

After starting to work out regularly and changing his diet, it took Dr. Will about five months to shed the punching belly. He weighed in around 218 pounds on his 5' 11.5" frame. His smart way of eating combined with his exercise regimen was reflected in his health as well. After his transformation, his cholesterol was only 160 mg/dl (normal in the United States is under 200), down from around 210.

Another turning point for Dr. Will was in June 2010 when his wife took a picture of him in the swimming pool. That picture showed him that his body was transformed—almost 50 pounds gone, and he was now ripped and chiseled.

**Dr. Success!**

As a result of his transformation, Dr. Will has gained more confidence, more energy for his kids and wife, more positivity, and a better outlook on life. Before Will started his exercise regime, his wife would often suggest that he find something that he enjoyed doing outside of work and family. Now, in addition to losing weight and feeling great, he has made a multitude of friends through various fitness communities and events, such as CrossFit, races, mud run competitions, and coaching other people. He's found his passion!

Dr. Will also connects the success of his transformation to his career and how he cares for patients. No longer sporting a big belly, he gives wellness advice, and people can see that he "walks the talk."

### Dr. Will's Current Regimen

Dr. Will loves working out. He exercises six days a week and has one recovery day where he stretches. He varies his workouts. Some days, he might do the Insanity DVD at home or run outside for five miles. If he goes to the gym, he might run on the treadmill, take a cardio class, or focus on body resistance training with pull-ups and push-ups. He exercises about one to one and a half hours a day.

# NuTricia's Takeaways

Good nutrition can help you feel great and decrease disease risk. It's the foundation of a healthy life. Moving up the nutrition staircase, whether it's one or several steps, can give you numerous healthy dividends, such as clearer skin, feeling better, and living a longer, more fulfilling life. One of the best things you can do for your health is to ensure that you are eating at least three different vegetables each day.

## Key Points to Remember

- Use the NuTricia's Great Plate as a simple visual reminder to eat a healthy, balanced diet.
- Keep climbing the nutrition staircase. It is a series of steps that never end.
- Stay out of Nutrition Jail! Do this by eating healthfully and watching for words such as "enriched" and "partially hydrogenated," which ultimately mean you are not getting optimal nutrition from the product you are buying!

# CHAPTER 2

# Smart Shopping

*Eat what grows from the ground, what falls*
*from the tree, and what swims in the sea.*

—Anthony Liberti, Sr., my grandfather

My grandfather may have been ahead of his time. Nutritionists agree that the healthiest diets are those predominantly made up of whole foods—those with minimal or no processing. Chips and candy wouldn't be found on my grandfather's list of things to eat! Some packaged foods can be included as part of a healthy diet, but the less processed food we eat, the healthier we are, and the longer we'll live. And research now is showing this!

In fact, a recent study of over 45,000 French adults found that just a 10 percent increase in the amount of ultra-processed foods eaten can be associated with a 14 percent increased mortality risk.[7] And in case you're wondering, mortality is a euphemism for dying. Yikes! Examples of foods that are considered ultra-processed are ready-to-heat, ready-to-eat foods as well as packaged snacks, bread, candies, processed foods, and sugary drinks.[8]

One way to avoid these ultra-processed foods and improve nutritional habits is by being a smart shopper, which involves learning the best way to shop for food. Several smart strategies can be employed when shopping to maximize nutrition.

## Dig Deep into the Food Label

In order to ensure a healthy, balanced diet, you need to know what you're eating. The best way to do that is to look carefully at food packaging. From ingredients to nutritional information to allergy warnings, there's a lot of information to be gleaned from the words on a package.

The food label is a great place to start to get a better sense of what is actually in the food you eat. The numbers are helpful, but the ingredient list is more telling. Ingredients are listed by weight—from highest to lowest. So, if you see something like sugar as the first ingredient (or even second or third), that's pretty revealing. It's probably a good idea to put that product down and keep looking.

Following are some tips and tricks for interpreting food labels that can help you quickly discern whether or not you should toss that food in your cart, or if it would be better to toss it out.

**US Food Label**

## Nutrition Facts

4 servings per container
**Serving size 1 1/2 cup (208g)**

Amount per serving
**Calories** **240**

| | % Daily Value* |
|---|---|
| **Total Fat** 4g | **5%** |
| Saturated Fat 1.5g | **8%** |
| Trans Fat 0g | |
| **Cholesterol** 5mg | **2%** |
| **Sodium** 430mg | **19%** |
| **Total Carbohydrate** 46g | **17%** |
| Dietary Fiber 7g | **25%** |
| Total Sugars 4g | |
| Includes 2g Added Sugars | **4%** |
| **Protein** 11g | |
| Vitamin D 2mcg | 10% |
| Calcium 260mg | 20% |
| Iron 6mg | 35% |
| Potassium 240mg | 6% |

* The % Daily Value (DV) tells you how much a nutrient in a serving of food contributes to a daily diet. 2,000 calories a day is used for general nutrition advice.

## Food Label Percentages

The Percent Daily Value (DV) column on the right-hand side of the food label tells you how much of a nutrient is provided per serving based on someone eating a 2,000 calorie diet. You can use this information to help decide whether or not to purchase the item or find another food instead. One food label trick I like to use relies on just three percentage numbers—5%, 10%, and 20%. Finding these numbers on a food label can help you quickly zero in on whether a nutrient is high or low in a specific food. Here's how it works:

- If the label lists 5% or lower for % DV, then the food is considered low in that nutrient. (If your chosen food is 2% saturated fat, then yay! But, if you're buying a grain-based product and it's only 2% fiber—yikes!)
- If the label lists 10% for the DV, then the food has a significant amount of that nutrient. That really just means a middle-of-the-road amount, not too much or too little of a specific nutrient.
- If the label lists 20% DV or more of a particular nutrient, then the food is considered to be relatively high in that nutrient. (If that's 30% calcium, then yay! But if that number shows the food contains 30% sodium—yikes!)
- In Canada, they simplify it even more with just two numbers to consider. If an ingredient is 5% or less, then the food is considered low in that nutrient, if it is 15% or higher, it's considered to have a lot of that nutrient.

Of course, these are meant to be guidelines to help you evaluate foods when shopping. Just because a food has a small (or large) amount of a particular nutrient doesn't mean it is or is not healthy. For example, a low percentage of fiber does not make milk unhealthy—you wouldn't expect to find a significant amount of fiber in dairy products.

But Daily Value percentages can give you a quick snapshot of the nutritional benefits or detriments of different foods. What follows are a few more tips and tricks to help you make sense of food labels and what's in your food.

## Sugar Calculation

You've probably heard that you need to watch your sugar intake, and this makes sugar another important ingredient to watch out for when shopping smart. The challenge is that it can be difficult to determine just how much sugar is in a food because the information is often presented in a way that's not easily understood.

Canada takes a great approach when listing sugar on food labels. The new Canadian food label groups all sugars contained in a food together, which gives consumers a pretty accurate idea of just how much total sugar a particular food contains. In comparison, the U.S. food label can be deceiving because multiple sources of sugar are listed separately on the label. If you added up the separately listed sugars, you might find that sugar is suddenly the first ingredient on the list, which is a good reason to put that product back.

It can also be difficult to figure out how much sugar is actually in a serving. Have you ever noticed that the amount of sugar in a food is listed in grams? For most of us, that measurement doesn't really mean anything. Can you picture the 29 grams of added sugar in the typical 1.69-ounce package of M&Ms? Probably not. But if I told you it was seven teaspoons of sugar, you might take notice.

Here's a simple formula to use when shopping to help you translate sugars listed in grams into teaspoons:

**Take Grams of Sugar and Divide by 4 to Get Teaspoons**

You can round up or down to keep the math easy. In the M&Ms example, I rounded 29 to 28, then divided 28 grams by 4 to get 7 teaspoons.

## American Heart Association Guideline for Added Sugar

Why worry about your sugar intake and this calculation? The American Heart Association has set the limit for added sugar to six teaspoons per day for women and nine teaspoons a day for men. For a woman, that one bag of M&Ms gets you there and then some. The American Heart Association limit may even be too high, especially for those who struggle with their weight. Optimally, I recommend that on most days, people aim for zero to three teaspoons of added sugar.

Luckily, beginning in January 2021, the FDA will require all packaged foods to use the new U.S. food label shown previously. In addition to using updated Daily Values and showing more realistic serving sizes, added sugar grams will be listed separately from total sugar.

So, for example, a popular cereal with sugar-coated raisins currently shows 13 grams of sugar on the label. It's hard to distinguish how many of the sugar grams occur naturally in the raisin (as nature intended) and how many have been added in the sugar coating. The newer label will identify the total grams of sugar in a serving and then separately list added sugars.

With the new label requirements, I believe some companies may begin to change the formulations of their products. Some may try to decrease added sugars, but others, I fear, would rather not tell you how much actual sugar is in their product. They may start using more sugar alcohols and artificial sugars.

I've seen this happening with a popular brand's chocolate chip granola bar. Previously, they did not contain sugar alcohols. Now, they have replaced some of the sugar with sugar alcohols. Sugar alcohols can be upsetting to the stomach and can have a laxative effect. Companies use them to lower the sugar content of their products because they offer sweetness with fewer calories than regular sugar.

## Calcium Trick

Calcium is vital for bone health—particularly for women (and especially as we age). Your doctor or dietitian may even have told you to try to consume a certain number of milligrams of calcium each day. An easy way to calculate milligrams can be done directly from the percentage DV listed on the label. Simply add a zero to the percentage, and you get the number of milligrams. For instance, if your yogurt says 25% calcium, add a "0" and you get 250 milligrams of calcium per serving.

## Sodium Comparison

An excellent trick for estimating if a food might be high in sodium is to compare the sodium milligrams per serving to the number of calories per serving. In general, you want the sodium number to be less than the calories.

For example, a **popular brand of tomato sauce contains** 460 milligrams of sodium per serving **and is 70** calories per serving. In this instance, the sodium milligrams are far higher than the calories, which suggests you should find a better sauce.

In contrast, another brand of tomato sauce that has no salt added contains only 40 milligrams of sodium per serving and is 50 calories per serving. Since the sodium milligrams are less than the calories, this is a better option.

## Tricia's Troublesome Twelve Food Additives

While there are over 3,000 additives listed as safe in the Food and Drug Association's database, I am going to highlight 12 pesky ones that you should try to avoid.[9] I think it's smart to avoid most additives if possible. Artificial sugars are additives to avoid as well, and they are discussed in Chapter 3.

Part of the FDA's mission is "ensuring the safety of our nation's food supply."[10] The FDA makes decisions about food additives based on testing conducted by the companies who developed the food additives and the results they submit to the FDA. This seems to be a conflict of interest because these companies are the ones who will make money when the additives are used in the food supply.

For instance, Thaumatin is a sweetener that may gain traction over the next few years. It is advertised as a sweetener that has been used for one hundred years and comes from the Katemphe plant in West Africa. It has GRAS (generally regarded as safe) status from the FDA, but that is based on documentation submitted by a company that will be manufacturing and selling Thaumatin.

It's eye opening to read about the intense #Frankenfood manufacturing process, outlined in the documentation submitted to the FDA to support the claim that their product is safe. The manufacturing process includes using bacteria to transfer genes from the Katemphe plant to genes in spinach or beet plants, which are then used to grow it. It is a bioengineered food where various chemicals can be used along the way to guide the process of producing the sweet Thaumatin. Consumers will think they are eating a clean low-calorie natural sweetener; however, they will actually be eating a substance that's highly processed and engineered.

The following is a list of twelve additives that I suggest you avoid. The descriptions cover how they are used in food production and/or the commonly listed names used on food labels.

## Troublemaker #1: Emulsifiers

**Uses:** Keep processed food ingredients together and dispersed evenly throughout (examples: polysorbate 80, soy lecithin).

Envision the picture perfect salad dressings on the supermarket aisle and compare that to the dressing you make at home. At home, the oil and vinegar separate, and the spices fall to the bottom. In the supermarket, the ingredients are held together in an emulsion. Emulsifiers work like a charm because they have water-loving and fat-loving components. The water-loving part can attach to watery substances, and the fat-loving part can stick to the fat. By holding these other substances together, the emulsifiers help create products that look tasty to eat. But they may cause problems under that pretty facade. #carnivalfood

When mice were given an amount of an emulsifier that's comparable to an acceptable amount for humans, they developed a variety of concerning issues, including inflammation, insulin resistance, increased food consumption, increased fat tissue, abnormal liver tests, and increased intestinal permeability.[11] When the emulsifier polysorbate 80 was compared with plantain and broccoli, it was found that the plantain and broccoli reduced the movement of E. coli bacteria across the microfold cells of the intestine, while polysorbate 80 increased the movement of E. coli across these cells. And, yes, you are correct if you are wondering if E. coli is that nasty bacteria that we don't want to get across our intestinal wall!

Soy lecithin is another junky ingredient used as an emulsifier in many foods, including nutrition bars, chocolate, salad dressings, margarine, and cooking sprays. It is extracted from soybeans — often using hexane.[12]

> ## How About Using a Natural Emulsifier Instead?
>
> Mustard is a natural emulsifier. A little bit of Dijon mustard with extra virgin olive oil, your favorite vinegar, and a spice mix creates a tasty dressing! By using at least one fresh herb in your salad, you can really wake up the flavor! You can even add in some cut-up fruit, so you don't have to add any sweetener to the dressing.

### Troublemaker #2: Hexane

**Use:** Extracts protein, oil, and lecithin from beans and seeds.

Hexane is a highly flammable industrial chemical distilled from petroleum. The European Union sets hexane residue limits on oils, flours, proteins, soy products, and cereal germ. In the U.S., when it comes to drugs, the FDA classifies it as one of the Class 2 solvents which "should be limited in pharmaceutical products because of their inherent toxicity."[13] However, for food, the FDA only sets limits on hexane residues for spices and hops.[14]

Hexane, a component of gasoline and jet fuel, is used as a solvent in the extraction of oils such as canola, soy, cottonseed, corn, flax, olive, peanut, sunflower, and safflower. It is used to remove isolated proteins from soy, which often show up in energy bars and powders. It is also used to extract fish protein, shea butter, and many flavors.[15]

If you use baby formula with DHA or ARA, it's important to check to see if these brain-boosting compounds were extracted using hexane. If they were, your baby's brain boost might really be a brain bust. There have been reports of babies having gastrointestinal complications due to hexane. I believe hexane should not be used to process any food ingredients—especially not food for infants![16] The FDA recently condoned the use of hexane-extracted canola lecithin in baby formula … of course, based on safety tests submitted by the manufacturer.[17]

The USDA says exposure to hexane may irritate the skin and eyes, inhalation may cause headaches as well as numbness in extremities, and ingestion may cause abdominal pain and nausea.[18] The Environmental Protection Agency (EPA) reports that chronic exposure to hexane is associated with neurotoxicity in rats.[19]

After hearing conflicting information about canola oil several years back, I decided to dig a little deeper to get the scoop on whether this omega-3 rich oil is good for you. I learned from a canola oil representative at a conference that it is processed with hexane. I immediately switched to organic canola oil. Before the switch, my husband found that his stomach was getting upset with the conventional canola oil. Once we switched to organic, his stomach no longer bothered him after eating it. I'm pretty convinced that it was hexane residues that were not working for him.

So, what can you do? Look for organic oils, extra virgin olive oil, organic protein isolates, organic flavor extracts, and organic lecithins. Also, look for the word "expeller-pressed" before the word oil in the ingredient list. This means the oil was extracted mechanically rather than through a solvent process. When it comes to purchasing oil, don't settle for less.

## Buyer Beware!

Companies often choose solvents to extract oils rather than the healthier mechanical extrusion techniques because they recover more oil with the solvent process. Solvent extractions are also cheaper, so from their view, more efficient. The companies claim that steam-processing removes the hexane. I'm not convinced.

**Troublemaker #3: Texturizers, Thickeners, and Fillers**

**Use:** Improves the texture and "mouth feel" of foods (examples maltodextrin and carrageenan).

Texturizers are compounds that improve the mouth feel of foods — adding creaminess, for example. Thickeners increase the volume of food. Maltodextrin can be added to cereals and snack foods to "improve" the texture, making them more crisp and shinier. Maltodextrin is used as a bulking agent in the artificial sugar Splenda. It can act as a carrier of flavors and juices in powdered form. Although it may make foods shinier, it may have a darker effect on your intestines. When studied as part of the ingredients in Splenda, maltodextrin has been found to negatively affect the intestinal health of mice with Crohn's disease.[20] The Splenda fed mice had an overgrowth of the yummy and delicious E. coli bacteria (Yes, I am using sarcasm here!).[21]

Carrageenan is used as a texturizer. You may see it in your ice cream or almond milk. It's also often found in candy, chocolate milk, coffee products, and dairy products. In 2016, the USDA took carrageenan off the list of acceptable ingredients for organic foods. This came after the research provided to the National Organics Standard Board proved that carrageenan causes inflammation and may be a carcinogen.

**Troublemaker #4: Propyl Gallate**

**Use:** Preservative.

Propyl gallate may be found in chewing gum, microwave popcorn, sausage, and lard. One research study concluded that "the consumption of propyl gallate as a food additive at a relatively high dose may induce toxicity and carcinogenicity."[22] Bakers have developed contact dermatitis from working with this food additive.[23]

Do you want to know another particularly unsavory use for propyl gallate? It is one of the ingredients allowed to be in those sticky labels that adhere to your fruit. I've always been leery of those labels and prefer to discard the area of the food that comes in contact with them. Do you want to be chewing on anything that may be toxic and carcinogenic?

## Troublemaker #5: Gums

**Use:** Added to thicken, texturize, emulsify and stabilize foods, and for the chew factor in chewing gum.

Have you noticed that gums are now included in many ingredient lists? Almost every salad dressing on the shelves in supermarkets includes xanthan gum. Additionally, most almond milk brands contain gellan gum. What are these gums? Shockingly, they are made from the dried up ooze secreted by bacteria that are fed sugar. The ooze is dried using isopropyl alcohol, and some residual alcohol is allowed in the final ingredient. These gums haven't been tested well.

Even ten or twenty years ago, gums were far less common additives. Our grandparents didn't grow or use these in family recipes. We are the lab rats! Have you signed up to be a lab rat? At least study subjects get paid. We are lab rats who are paying to be part of the gruesome gum experiment.

The other gum that's troublesome is the chewing gum you may be chomping on as you read this book. Most chewing gum is a scary witch's brew of ingredients. On the ingredient list for gum, there's an ingredient called gum base. Dig a little deeper into FDA records, and you'll find that gum base may contain synthetic human made rubber type materials. Plasticizer chemicals are used to make the substance chewy. Besides gum base, many gums contain artificial flavor, artificial sugars, sugar alcohols, and preservatives. Just an FYI, we never learned in dietetics schooling how the body digests and absorbs human made rubber materials. Just sayin'.

> Julie Hylinski Myers gave up her gum after hearing my session at a conference in Florida. Two weeks later, she noticed that the headaches she'd had her whole adult life had gone away. Now that's a healthy dividend!

### Troublemaker #6: Propylparaben

**Use:** Added as an antimicrobial preservative.

Propylparaben is a synthetic, antimicrobial preservative that is found in food coloring, some tortillas, and other processed foods. It may negatively impact fertility. It may also contribute to breast tumor growth and breast cancer—just another reason to avoid products that contain food coloring.[24]

### Troublemaker #7: Artificial Colors

**Use:** Enhance appearance of foods Some common artificial colors are Yellow #5, Yellow #6, Red #40, Blue #1, and Blue #2.

Artificial colors often come from coal tar. In the European Union, several colors are required to have a warning on the label of the food they are found in, stating that they may affect attention and activity. These aren't the only troublesome colors.

In addition to being added to candy, soft drinks, and baked goods, Blue #1 is also an ingredient in hair dye. Both Blue #1 and Blue #2 may be associated with cancer. Yuck! One of the compounds that is used as an ingredient in Red #40 caused cancer in animals.[25]

## No Sleep for the Silvermans!

It happened twice, only a few months apart. My son ate candy with artificial coloring and was wide awake in the middle of the night when he is usually sound asleep. When we put two and two together, we realized the candy—and I suspect the yellow dyes, in particular—are what kept him awake.

### Troublemaker #8: Artificial Flavors

**Use:** Added to make food more flavorful and tasty. Many artificial flavors don't have to be listed individually by name on a product label (and are often comprised of a combination of chemicals).

One of the problems with artificial flavors is that the companies who make them are the ones who conduct tests to determine if they are safe. This seems to be a massive conflict of interest. Another issue is that food labels don't have to list individual flavor names, which keeps you in the dark. Avoid buying products that contain artificial flavors as an ingredient.

The Center for Science in the Public Interest (CSPI) and other health advocacy groups sued the FDA in 2018 to get seven flavoring ingredients banned due to their carcinogenic properties (benzophenone, ethyl acrylate, methyl eugenol, myrcene, pulegone, pyridine, and styrene).[26] This pressure worked, and the FDA no longer allows these flavors to be used.

### Troublemaker #9: BHT and BHA

**Use:** Added as preservatives and found in many packaged foods as well as chewing gum.

BHT and BHA preservatives are banned in the European Union but are still allowed in the U.S. and Canada. You can find BHT in crackers, cereal, chewing gum, and lots of other processed foods. BHA is not as common as BHT but can be found in dehydrated potato products, dried fruit, breakfast cereals, and other processed foods.

**Troublemaker #10: Nitrates, Nitrites, and Celery Powder**

**Use:** Added in concentrated form as preservatives and colorants.

Sodium nitrites and nitrates appear on the *avoid list* on CSPI's chemical cuisine website.[27] They are associated with cancer. What's troublesome is that food companies have gotten the message that people are trying to avoid nitrates and nitrites, so now many are switching to celery powder. While it sounds natural, celery powder also contains nitrates which turn into nitrosamines in your body that may have carcinogenic effects.

**Troublemaker #11: Phosphates**

**Use:** Added as preservatives, acidifying agents, acidity buffers, emulsifying agents, stabilizers, taste intensifiers, and also to reduce the clumpiness of powders.[28]

Phosphates are contained in soda and many processed foods. They are often listed as phosphoric acid. They impart flavor and protect against the growth of microorganisms.

Phosphates in natural foods aren't the problem since naturally occurring ones don't get completely absorbed. The problem lies in phosphate additives which raise serum phosphate levels in people with advanced chronic kidney disease. Phosphates can cause vascular damage, such as endothelial dysfunction and vascular calcification.[29]

Many soda drinkers drink their way into diabetes. With continued consumption, they can end up with kidney disease and may eventually need dialysis. Many people on dialysis are finally told they can't drink soda due to the phosphates. Why not tell everyone not to drink soda *now*? Then, they can kick those cans of poison away for good!

## Troublemaker #12: Aluminum

**Use:** Added to baking powders to maintain consistency.

My biggest beef with aluminum is that it may play a role in Alzheimer's disease. China has banned some aluminum containing ingredients. Where do we see a lot of it? In baking powder. So, when you eat processed baked goods, you might be getting served some aluminum. If you are doing the baking, choose aluminum free baking powders.

These are just 12 of many food additives that plague processed foods. Your best bet for creating healthy dividends is to eat the least amount of processed foods possible.

There's another sneaky substance to be aware of—acrylamide. It isn't an additive and is not on any ingredient list, but it may be in the food you're eating. Acrylamide forms when you take a carbohydrate-rich food and heat it to a very high temperature. It's in bread, crackers, potato chips, and French fries. And don't get angry at the messenger for telling you this— roasted coffee beans also have acrylamide. The World Health Organization has been warning countries to get the word out about acrylamide. I heard it making some buzz in the news several years back but haven't heard much buzz lately. You are getting this info now, so use it well. Stay away from burnt toast and the items above because acrylamide has been associated with cancer in animals.

> ## What's in Your Bread?
>
> Remember Caster Salemi, the 97-year-old dynamo? One thing I found very fascinating about him is that he doesn't eat store-bought bread. He goes to a bakery to get fresh bread. Take a look at your bread label. You will most likely see a very long list of ingredients with many additives and preservatives. Since bread is a staple food for many people, why not make these staple foods as healthy as possible? I recommend organic breads. Some organic breads are in the frozen section of the supermarket to extend shelf life since they don't contain preservatives.

To learn about other additives to avoid and for more shopping tips, be sure to follow me at Facebook.com/TriciaSilverman. I periodically post videos when I'm in the supermarket and have helpful tips to share.

## Other Packaging Information

In addition to the nutritional information and ingredient lists discussed above, product packaging can also provide you with details about the source of ingredients and how they have been grown or processed. But buyer beware—some of the packing information can be misleading.

For instance, I suggest watching out when products are labeled with the word "smart." You and I can mix up sugar, flour, and every lousy additive mentioned above, and then slap a label that says smart on the packaging to make people think it is healthy. I think your best bet for creating healthy dividends is to invest most in foods that don't have labels … your vegetables and fruits!

## Genetically Modified Food

The World Health Organization defines genetically modified foods as "foods derived from organisms whose genetic material (DNA) has been modified in a way that does not occur naturally, e.g., through the introduction of a gene from a different organism."[30] I recommend avoiding GMO foods whenever possible. We are the lab rats for the big GMO experiment. Ingredients derived from corn, soy, canola, and sugar beet are often GMO unless they are listed as organic.[31]

One of the problems with some genetically modified ingredients is that they are modified to be resistant to Roundup®, a commonly used weed killer, which has glyphosate as its principal ingredient. Genetically modified soybeans have been shown to have high levels of glyphosate.[32] Unfortunately, other crops such as wheat, oats, and beans, are often targeted with glyphosate before harvest. In 2016, the FDA did a glyphosate analysis. It reported, "Non-violative levels of glyphosate were found in 173 (63.1%) of the corn samples and 178 (67.0%) of the soybean samples and non-violative levels of glufosinate were found in 4 (1.4%) of the corn samples and 3 (1.1%) soybean samples."[33]

Perhaps the benchmarks for what violative levels are should be questioned, especially since there have been two recent cases that have been ruled in favor of cancer-stricken people who have sued the makers of Roundup® because they developed cancer after exposure to glyphosate. Choosing organic foods can help prevent unnecessary exposure to glyphosate and other pesticides in our foods.

## Organic vs. Nonorganic

People often ask if it's worth the extra cost to buy organic? The short answer is that it depends on the product. When it comes to fresh produce, the Environmental Working Group (EWG) has come up with their list of the Dirty Dozen™ foods. For these fruits and vegetables, whenever possible, you should choose the organic variety due to the high level of pesticide residues on conventional versions. The "dirty" top three are strawberries, spinach, and kale. The EWG also developed the Clean Fifteen™ list which outlines 15 foods that are safe to buy conventional (many of these have skins we don't eat like bananas). The clean top three are avocados, sweet corn, and pineapple. Go to EWG.org to get the full lists which are updated annually.

When you see USDA organic seal, it means that at least 95% of the ingredients are organic. The remaining ingredients may be nonorganic because they are not available as organic, or they are ingredients that are not yet on the USDA's National List. If you see the organic seal, and there is language on the label that says 100% organic, then you can assume this is true. If the label says, "Made with Organic," then at least 70% of the ingredients are organic.[34]

So, to answer the question of whether or not you should buy organic—if your finances allow, I think going organic for most of your foods is an excellent idea. If not, use the lists from Environmental Working Group to help guide your purchases. If you need to purchase primarily conventional fruits and vegetables, try to buy the bulk of your produce from the Clean 15 list. It's a good idea to rinse all produce thoroughly. Even if you can't buy organic, if you choose less processed, whole foods, you can limit your exposure to most of the #FrankenChemicals used to process food.

## Wild vs. Farm-Raised?

You can probably guess what I am going to say here, but in case you are still wondering—when buying fish, if you can afford wild, I think that's the way to go. Wild fish are raised in their natural environment, eating the foods that nature intended. Salmon, for example, are carnivores. They eat shrimp and krill, which provide natural astaxanthin (this gives salmon its signature color). With farmed salmon, a colorant may be added to make it look more like the wild fish. Farmed fish are forced to be omnivores: eating soy, corn, etc. in addition to fish. If wild fish is too expensive, you are still okay eating farmed fish. You'll still get a lean protein with a dose of healthy omega-3 fatty acids.

## Supermarket Shopping Strategies

Many people often complain that eating healthy costs too much. There's a little secret that lies in the shelf labels in your supermarket that can save you boatloads of money over your lifetime. That secret is unit pricing.

Unit pricing is the price per unit, such as the price per ounce or pound. It allows you to figure out what is the best price for the actual food you are buying regardless of the container size. You can use unit pricing to compare different sizes and/or brands of healthy foods, as well as paper products, and many other items you buy in the supermarket.

As a poor dietetic intern, I was trying to manage my limited funds. I would buy the largest box of Cheerios, assuming it was the cheapest, and I would stuff it sideways into the one cabinet I had in my tiny kitchen. The cabinet door wouldn't shut, and the box would be partially hanging out, but I didn't mind because I was saving money. Or was I?

One day, I grabbed my home economics textbook from college, and flipped to a chapter I had never read before about unit pricing. It resulted in one of those aha moments you sometimes have in your life. I couldn't believe no one had ever told me about this. Before this discovery, I would occasionally use my calculator to figure out the best price. Now, I simply use unit pricing to find the best deal, and it's right on the shelf label.

Let's take a closer look at unit pricing. The example below comes from the USDA website and shows different pricing for different product sizes.[35]

If you buy the 32-ounce yogurt, the shelf price is $1.62, but the price per unit is $.05 per ounce. For the 6-ounce yogurt, the price you pay is $.72, but the unit price is $.12 per ounce. You are paying double the price per ounce when you buy the smaller container.

After I learned about unit pricing, I found that sometimes the medium box of cereal was cheaper, and it would fit better in my one cabinet, as well!

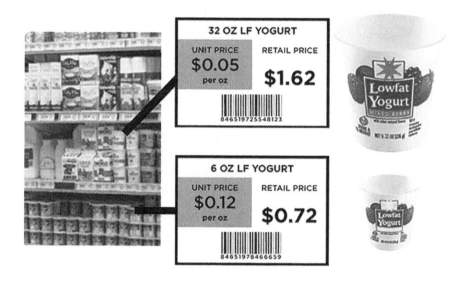

## Other Food Shopping Tips

As you make your grocery run, there are some things to remember to help ensure you make healthy choices.

- **Don't Shop Hungry.** You've heard this one before. Before you go shopping, try to have a meal or a healthy snack (such as a 100 calorie pack of almonds or other nuts). When shopping hungry, people tend to make more impulse purchases and poorer choices. But what about those times when you can't avoid shopping hungry? First, opt for the candy-free checkout aisle if your store has one. The following items can quickly and healthfully satisfy your hunger when you get in the car:
  - Single-serve yogurt (There are often utensils available near the salad bar or checkout. Just ask. Or, you can buy a small box of spoons. I keep a bag of disposable utensils in my car.)
  - Banana or orange
  - Fruit salad
  - Salad bar items
  - Individual packet of nuts, roasted soybeans, or roasted chickpeas
- **Shop the Perimeter, and Shop for a Rainbow of Produce.** The fresh foods (produce, fish/poultry, dairy, etc.) tend to be situated on the outside aisles (perimeter) of most grocery stores. If you stick to these, you'll likely end up with the healthiest purchases. Make sure you are spending enough time in the produce aisle, and you select a variety of colorful fruits and vegetables (a rainbow). This area of the supermarket has the most profound influence on your health.
- **Stay Away From the Snack Food and Soda Aisles.** These are usually found in the center of the supermarket. To avoid

temptation, remember the tip mentioned above, and stay in areas of the store—usually the perimeter—where foods are fresher and have less junky ingredients and chemicals added.

- **Shop Local When You Can.** It seems like the further food is shipped, the higher the likelihood it will contain something unsavory. For instance, some fruit is picked early, then sprayed with ethylene gas to get it to ripen on its journey to the consumer. Consider shopping at local farm stands or even buying a share from a CSA (Community Supported Agriculture) group. A CSA share typically entitles you to a share of the crops of a farm for a specified number of weeks. Go to LocalHarvest.org to find a farmer's market or CSA opportunity near you.

- **Avoid Convenience Stores as Much as Possible.** I call these vice stores. This is where it's easy to get a sugar, alcohol, cigarette, and gambling fix. Sure, there are healthier options. But you'll likely have to walk by the candy, chips, and soda. If you must go in, I would seek out the nuts, seeds, yogurt, and fruit.

## Produce Shelf Life Guide

If you would like to minimize the shopping trips per week (maybe only make one?), then planning becomes essential. When figuring out your meals for the week, plan to use your hardy vegetables and fruits (things like cabbage and apples) for meals later in the week. The following chart shows the approximate shelf life of some popular produce to help with meal planning.

**Produce that can last up to a week or longer.**

These are just guidelines. Use your best judgment, and when in doubt, throw it out.

## Fruits

Apples: 3 weeks

Citrus Fruits (oranges, grapefruit, lemons, limes): 2 weeks

Cranberries: 1 week

Grapes: 1 week

Kiwi: 10 days

Melons: 1 week

Pears: 3-10 days unripened, then 3-5 days when ripened

Pineapple: 1 week

## Vegetables

Artichokes: 1 week

Beets: 1-2 weeks

Bell Peppers: 1 week

Bok Choy: 1 week

Brussels Sprouts: 1 week

Cabbage: 2 weeks

Carrots: 2 weeks

Celeriac: 2 weeks

Celery: 1 week

Cucumber: 1 week

Fennel: 1 week

Lettuce: 1 week

Onions: 2 weeks in a cool, dry area

Parsnips: 1–2 weeks

Potatoes: 3 weeks in a cool, dark area

Radishes: 7–10 days

Rutabaga: 2 weeks

Sweet Potato: 10 days, not in refrigerator

Turnip: 1 week

Winter Squash: Several weeks at room temperature

## NuTricia's Takeaways

It's important to shop smarter to earn the dividends of feeling better and living longer. To limit your exposure to food additives and pesticides, choose foods that have a simple and very short ingredient list. Go organic when you can.

Here are some key takeaways from the chapter.

- Use the food label tricks to compare nutrients.
- Read through ingredient lists and avoid foods that contain ingredients you are unable to identify.
- Shop for a rainbow, and spend a large proportion of your shopping trip in the produce section.

# CHAPTER 3

# Reducing Sugar

Limiting your sugar consumption is one of the best things you can do for your health—literally from head to toe. You'll lower your risk for many chronic diseases, including diabetes, heart disease, and cancer. You're also likely to reduce excess fat on your body while improving how you feel and think.

## Sugar and Chronic Diseases

Recent research indicates that sugar can have serious effects on your brain. It may increase your risk for Alzheimer's, and it may also affect the hippocampus area, which is associated with memory.[36] It may decrease your brain volume.

Sugar also rots your teeth and can diminish the effectiveness of your immune system. A participant in one of my programs told me about being alarmed by a wound that wouldn't heal. She read up on refined sugar, cut it from her diet, and the wound healed.

Sugar also affects our blood. It's associated with the metabolic syndrome and raises blood pressure—a notion most doctors don't even know about. Sugar also can raise blood triglycerides and lower the levels of HDL cholesterol (the "H for Healthy" cholesterol). That's the number you want to see on the higher side, as opposed to LDL cholesterol (the "L for Lousy"), which you want to stay low.

A junky diet with too much sugar can lead to diabetes. Uncontrolled diabetes can be devastating and lead to neuropathies—damage that affects the nerve endings in your eyes, toes, and other parts of your body.

During a clinical rotation of my dietetic internship, I learned about debridement, a procedure I had never heard of until then. A patient with advanced diabetes had a wound on his foot that would not heal. The odor that results from debridement (scraping away the damaged tissue) is an unforgettable stench that you never want to have to smell in your life—ever. Unfortunately for this poor soul, this procedure was unsuccessful, and they needed to amputate below the knee.

Experiences like this helped clarify my conviction that I wanted to help people way before they found themselves at this end stage of health. I wanted to work with people to help them understand the dangers of eating poorly, and the benefits of making good choices.

## Sugar and Your Waistline

Sugar can widen your waistline, which puts more pressure on your knees and joints, and is associated with gout.

I met an attendee at a health fair who held a prominent position in her town. She was in her 70s and had lost over 20 pounds simply by giving up sugar. This demonstrates the hidden impact sugar can have on your diet (and waistline), but it also shows that you can lose weight at any age — especially when you find the source of your weight struggles.

Another person I met at one of my employee wellness programs cut out after-dinner desserts (often a big source of sugar) and went from prediabetes to no sign of diabetes at all. She shared that a bonus is that her clothes fit her better, particularly in the belly area.

## Limiting Sugar Helps to Reveal Your Muscles

"I followed your advice about the sugary drinks, and this year, I lost five belt loops." This is what Josh Robinson, an online fitness coach from Collierville, Tennessee, told me when I saw him at the 2018 Atlanta SCW Fitness Education Convention. I had first met him at the same conference the previous year when he attended one of my sessions titled, "Sugar Shockers and Shakedown."

Josh is a former police officer, and even as a personal trainer, he still loved honeybuns, Reese's Pieces, and sugary drinks. He decided to give up most added sugar for 12 weeks. For the first two weeks, he had lots of sugar cravings. His mouth was watering, and he was dreaming about honeybuns. To help get him through, he carried a lot of fruit around with him to eat when he craved something sweet. He also drank two glasses of water two to three times per day. His cravings stopped in three weeks.

Along with sugar, he avoided fried food, bread, and alcohol. In 12 weeks, he lost 10 pounds and four belt loops. He noticed he had fewer headaches, relief from his bursitis, increased energy and attention, and less frequent mood swings.

Fast forward one year. Josh hit a couple of bumps along the road. His dog died, and the emotional toll made it harder for him to stay focused and disciplined. He slid back into his old habits and gained back some of the weight.

Josh decided to do a wellness challenge, along with his personal training clients. This time, he gave up sugar **and** processed foods, while incorporating 30-minute workouts three to five days of the week. As a result, he lost 25 pounds and five notches on his belt in just over eight weeks. His muscles became more defined (particularly noticeable in his abs).

His results show that when looking to improve muscle tone, it's essential to combine both exercise and a decrease in sugar consumption to get the best results.

When I spoke with him after his initial weight loss in 2017, he mentioned that although he dropped a whopping array of processed foods and sugar from his diet, he was still drinking one energy drink per day, which had added sugar. The following year, as a result of our conversation, he gave that up too.

Here are Josh's before and after pictures, demonstrating the success of his most recent wellness challenge.

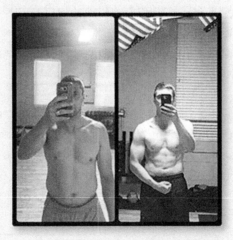

## How Much Sugar to Eat

Now, before you run from fruit because it has sugar, remember that eating fruit is one of the investments that will give you phenomenal healthy dividends, including cancer prevention and immune protection. Any fad diet that tells you to stop eating fruit is doing a disservice to your body and immune system. It's the **added sugar** that we need to avoid, not the sugar in whole foods, such as fresh fruit.

As mentioned in chapter 2, the American Heart Association has given us a helpful guideline for managing added sugars. It suggests that women limit their added sugar consumption to six teaspoons per day, and men limit it to nine teaspoons a day. I recommend setting your limit even lower than this. Why? First, because it's pretty clear that added sugars can quickly add unwanted weight. But also, if you are taking in significant amounts of added sugar, that most likely means you are consuming more processed foods. We've discussed all the unhealthy ingredients that can come along with these types of foods. For many people, the more sugar they eat, the more they crave it.

Watching your added sugar intake in teaspoons is a great way to start paying more attention to your diet. Remember the quick calculation to figure this out? To get teaspoons of sugar in a serving, take the number of grams listed on the label and divide this number by four. The resulting number tells you how many teaspoons of sugar are in a serving. I recommend aiming for three teaspoons or less of added sugar per day. Occasional indulgences with higher amounts of sugar can be planned as part of a healthy, enjoyable life. The key is to keep it low most of the time.

| Other Names for Added Sugar | |
| --- | --- |
| Brown rice syrup | Honey |
| Brown sugar | Invert sugar |
| Confectioner's sugar | Lactose |
| Cane sugar | Maltose |
| Corn sweetener | Malt syrup |
| Corn syrup | Maple syrup |
| Dextrin | Molasses |
| Dextrose | Palm Sugar |
| Evaporated cane juice | Raw sugar |
| Fructose | Sucanat |
| Fruit juice concentrates | Sucrose |
| Glucose | Sugar |
| High fructose corn syrup | Turbinado sugar |

Stevia and monk fruit are popular sweeteners that don't add calories and aren't artificial, but I still don't recommend daily use of them. I've found that I needed several packets of monk fruit sweetener to get any appreciable sweetness, and dextrose (corn sugar) is often added as an ingredient to monk fruit based sweeteners, which means you're still consuming added sugars. And a popular brand of stevia adds sugar alcohol which can give you an upset stomach or intestinal discomfort. An interesting study found that when beverages sweetened with monk fruit, stevia, or aspartame were compared to beverages sweetened with sugar, they all led to raised blood sugar and insulin after a test meal.[37]

## Sugar and Brain Fog

If you drastically cut back on your refined sugar (also known as added sugar) for a few weeks, I bet you will notice how much more clearly you think. I have seen this effect in myself—I am always more productive when my sugar intake is in control. I have surveyed attendees in my programs after the holidays, and they always note how much better they feel when they get back to more healthful eating after the holidays.

Sugar sweetened beverages are also associated with cognitive decline, so giving up the sugar may give you the healthy dividends of preserving your mental functioning as you age, and helping to prevent against dementia.[38]

## Sugar and Your Teeth

If you're worried about cavities and want strong teeth, avoiding refined sugar is one of the best things you can do. There is a known link between sugar and tooth decay. A healthy diet and regular brushing and flossing should keep your teeth in good condition. Remember the Hunzan culture we talked about before? In addition to having good eyesight, they also have great teeth. Dr. Banik noted this and attributed it to their healthy diet with no refined sugar.

# Artificial Sugars

Artificial sugars have been associated with cancer in animals. Diet soda (which contains artificial sugar) has been associated with dementia and strokes, as well as with heart attacks.[39] Many people report headaches with the consumption of aspartame.

Research has found that people tend to make up the calories they save when drinking diet soda by eating more at meals and snacks. Also, artificial sweeteners are so much sweeter than natural sugar that they may affect your taste buds, altering your perception of sweetness. Those healthy fruits don't taste as sweet anymore. I recommend reducing your consumption of artificial sugars, with the eventual goal of cutting them entirely from your diet.

> ## Common Artificial Sweeteners
>
> - Acesulfame Potassium (or Acesulfame-K)
> - Aspartame
> - Equal
> - Neotame
> - Saccharin
> - Sweet and Low
> - Sucralose (Splenda)

## Sugar Alcohol

Sugar alcohols are carbohydrates that are lower in calories because they don't get digested very well. They can upset the stomach and cause a laxative effect, especially if eaten in excess. They often appear in foods whose labels say sugar-free or low sugar. Two ladies from an employee wellness site told me that, after working together for over 20 years, they had never experienced the pain and discomfort that followed the shared eating of a bag of sugar-free jellybeans.

Your best bet is to avoid these nuisance ingredients. The easiest way to recognize these troublemakers is that they mostly end with the letters -itol.

> ## Sugar Alcohol Names
>
> - Sorbitol
> - Erythritol
> - Mannitol
> - Isomalt
> - Xylitol
> - Hydrogenated Starch Hydrolysates
> - Maltitol
> - Glycerol
> - Maltitol Syrup
> - Lactitol

# Reduce Your Sugar and Junk-Food Cravings

Cravings for sugary and junky foods often lead to the consumption of those foods, so it's important to prevent and reduce the cravings. The following 12 tips and tricks can help you get through these cravings. Know that giving up sugar gets easier with time and may take a few weeks.

## 12 Tips to Reduce Cravings

1. Reduce, limit, or avoid added sugar.
2. Keep tempting foods away, and move away from tempting foods.
3. Eat mindfully.
4. Reduce stress.
5. Aim for 7 to 9 hours of sleep.
6. Eat a balanced, healthy diet.
7. Make sure you are eating enough protein,
8. Plan your meals, snacks, and indulgences ahead of time.
9. Eat when you are hungry and don't wait until you're ravenous to eat, plan, or shop.
10. Don't go too long without eating. Eat roughly every 3 to 4 hours.
11. Drink water. Sometimes we think we are hungry when we may just need water.
12. When craving something sweet, reach for fruit.

## Chocolate Craving Hacks

Chocolate is a trigger for many people. You may have heard that chocolate contains antioxidants and can actually be good for you. This is true for dark (not milk) chocolate. Know that the junky food additive, soy lecithin, is in almost every chocolate bar on the market. We all know how hard it can be to stop eating things we love (like chocolate) once we start.

There are some things you can try when you get that urge to eat chocolate! These adaptations are meant to help you keep what you consume more healthful, and less likely to lead to eating too much. These are my favorite ways to get the taste of chocolate without indulging in candy.

1. Add one teaspoon of unsweetened cocoa to hot mint herbal tea.
2. Make energy balls with dates, unsweetened cocoa, and your favorite nuts. Mix in a food processor adding a little water as needed, and shape into balls with your hands. Place in the freezer for storage.
3. Sprinkle a teaspoon of unsweetened cocoa over organic frozen sweet dried cherries.
4. Add a teaspoon of unsweetened cocoa to your favorite smoothie recipe.

## Snacking Alternatives

The more sugar you eat and the more sugary beverages you drink, the more you will crave sugar. Here are some ideas for snacks that don't have added sugar. I recommend decreasing the amount of soda and diet soda consumed, and then switching over to chilled, carbonated water, preferably adding a squeeze of fresh lemon or lime to give flavor. Of course the best choice for a beverage is nature's choice: plain water.

## Low/No Added Sugar Snack Ideas

- Veggies and hummus or guacamole, or part-skim ricotta/lower-fat cottage cheese. Veggies: celery, carrots, cucumber, jicama, daikon (Japanese radish) peppers, broccoli, fennel, etc.

- Roasted soy nuts or chickpea snacks

- Greek or regular nonfat/lower fat plain yogurt with nut butter or nuts/seeds, and perhaps some fruit

- Broth-based veggie and bean soups

- Kale chips (see recipe at JoyBauer.com)

- Reduced fat cheese sticks

- Hard-boiled eggs or egg whites

- Scrambled eggs or egg whites with spinach

- Peanut butter or almond butter with celery sticks

- Nut butter with fruit

- Nuts and seeds

- Whole Foods Muesli cereal with milk

- Fruit – alone or with nuts or nut butter

- Brown rice cakes with reduced fat cheese

- Oatmeal with peanut butter or other add-ons: plain Greek yogurt, cut fruit, pumpkin pie spice, etc.

## NuTricia's Takeaways

Your investment in lowering the added sugar in your diet will lead to the healthy dividends of a lower risk for diabetes, heart disease, cancer, and Alzheimer's disease. You'll think more clearly, and if you're looking for weight loss, your clothes may become looser! Here are some key points:

- Cut your added sugar grams down to zero to three teaspoons per day.
- Four grams of sugar is equal to one teaspoon of sugar. When you see added sugar grams on the label, divide the grams by 4 to get the number of teaspoons.
- Cut down, then cut out artificial sugars, as they may lead to heart attacks, strokes, cancer, and dementia.
- Choose fruit when craving something sweet.

# CHAPTER 4

# Smart Dining Out

Meeting friends for dinner is a great way to connect and relax—good food, good friends, and no cleanup! But it may make you nervous if you're trying to establish new eating habits. You've done the hard work and are following your new nutrition plan at home, but it can be tough to make good choices at a restaurant.

Eating healthy doesn't mean you can never eat out. While the less you dine out, the easier it is to control your weight, sometimes it just happens, and it's best to have a few strategies so that you make good choices.

## Challenges When Dining Out

Years ago, I worked with a gentleman who had a high-ranking job in his community. He lived alone and dined out for literally every meal. He had no food in his house, and this lifestyle had been going on for years. Can you guess what health issues he had? High cholesterol, high blood pressure, and obesity, to name a few. His was an extreme case, but it showed me how living on a dine-out diet can take away your health.

The two biggest challenges you'll face when eating out are portion sizes and excessively high-calorie meals. Additionally, many meals contain hidden amounts of sugar, salt, and other lousy ingredients that create a witch's brew of future health concerns.

This reminds me of a time I was at a street fair in my town and trying to make a healthy food choice. There was plenty of pizza, ice cream, candy, and sausages to go around. I was thrilled to see a booth offering grilled chicken sandwiches. I ordered one and watched as they made the sandwiches. They toasted the bread perfectly, then took what looked like a large container that would typically hold ketchup or salad dressing and squeezed a ball of something onto the roll.

The substance immediately vanished into the bread. I asked them what mystery sauce was in the container, and they told me it was a butter sauce. The sandwich tasted great, but if I hadn't watched them make it, I would have assumed it was just a tasty, healthy sandwich. Unfortunately, with all that butter, I would hesitate to call it healthy. That taught me to be more cautious when ordering "healthy" foods. Now, I ask what types of sauces and extras are being used when I'm ordering.

Restaurants aren't the only danger zone. Meeting for coffee brings its own hazards. I consider the amount of sugar contained in some specialty coffees at a popular donut shop to be reckless. It's diabetes in a cup. One large frozen coffee specialty drink has over 800 calories and 187 grams of sugar. If you divide the sugar grams by four, you get 46.75 teaspoons of sugar in a large size. Who could even eat that much sugar alone? No one. But, everyone can easily down a beverage that disguises it with clever marketing and a carnival-like aesthetic.

Even when ordering simple coffee and tea drinks, it pays to pay attention. During my first job, I often ordered tea at the same popular donut shop. I bought the same brand of tea as the shop, but somehow my tea never tasted as good as what I bought at the shop. One day, I realized why, as I watched them pour milk into the drink. I had always assumed they put in maybe a few tablespoons of milk, but this was closer to almost a cup. They were pouring in around 80 more calories than I was calculating.

Additionally, at home, I only added a small amount of skim milk. That explained the better taste at the donut shop, and I realized that the eighty extra calories a day would equal eight pounds over the year. I stopped buying my tea out after that.

# Make a Plan

Since calories and out of control portions sizes are issues with restaurants, you need to have a game plan before heading out the door. Here are things to keep in mind.

### Check menus

Instead of arriving at a restaurant unsure of what's on the menu, go online, and look at the menu before you leave. This may even change your mind about which restaurant you visit. I'll never forget how shocked a participant at one of my seminars was after seeing how many calories were in the chicken parmesan (her favorite dish) at a local restaurant chain.

### Create your own smaller portion

Consider ordering the small or kid-size meal. When this isn't an option, I suggest dividing the meal in half and packing up the other half to take home. Packing the food to take with you can be very helpful; this way, you are not tempted to eat it. Ask for a to-go container when you first order. This makes cleanup easier for the waitstaff.

## Quality over quantity

Another way to control portions is to eat for quality rather than quantity. Look into where your food was grown or raised. Pick restaurants that cook from scratch and use local ingredients. Some restaurants grow their own herbs or have agreements with local farms. Juice bars often use very healthy ingredients that they put in their juices, salads, acai bowls, and smoothies.

## Look for healthier restaurants

In addition to juice bars, healthier restaurants can be found by looking for vegetarian restaurants and ethnic restaurants. When traveling, I like to look for Asian restaurants because I know I can always get a pile of fresh steamed vegetables as part of my meal. I often pair this with steamed chicken or steamed tofu, and brown rice with ginger sauce on the side.

I also like the salad chains and quick Mexican chains that have popped up. You can get fresh, tasty food fast in these restaurants. I have found nice vegetarian options at Indian restaurants, as well. One of my favorites is chana masala, a chickpea dish with onions, tomatoes, and yummy spices (including one of my favorite spice mixes—garam masala).

## Order with consideration

One thing that's important to remember when dining out is that the food has been created to taste good. Just because it doesn't taste too sweet or too salty, doesn't mean a ton of sugar and salt haven't been used. Restaurants are in business to make food taste great. I learned this firsthand when I was consulting with a restaurant. The chefs were making risotto, and they went through several rounds of adding salt, cream, and butter until they determined it was worthy of their customers. After viewing how much of these ingredients they added, I thought it would taste too buttery and salty. But it didn't. It was the best risotto I've eaten to this day! Your taste buds may not be as discerning as you think!

This is one of the problems with restaurant food. Chefs are fantastic at developing flavor experiences that delight your taste buds, so you keep going back to the same restaurant over and over again. Don't make the mistake of thinking that since the food doesn't taste salty, that they're not adding a lot of salt. They probably are.

With that in mind, be thoughtful when ordering. Ask what the soup and vegetable of the day are. These can be healthy options, especially if they are non-starchy vegetables, and vegetable or bean-based soups. Avoid saucy, cheesy, and fried choices. Sauces are often filled with extra sodium and calories, cheese is loaded with saturated fat, and the fried options often double the calories of their unfried counterparts.

I used to advise people to avoid the croutons but didn't explain the *why* behind my reasoning. After taking a cooking class where we made croutons, I can now say with great certainty that they should be avoided because they are loaded with sodium, and provide a fast track to a bloated and puffy body.

## Simplify with Go-To Choices

Think about having a few go-to options that you can reliably order from just about any menu. Having these healthy meal selections in mind can help you navigate a menu more quickly and healthily.

On days when you may be too stressed, tired, or sick to make food on your own, you may want to pick up a quick meal. Every area has its spots. For instance, in the Boston suburb area where I live, my go-to's for faster meals are Fresh City, Chipotle, SweetGreen, Honeygrow, and Asian restaurants. I have my favorite meals ready to order at each. For other restaurants, my go-to healthy meal is a salad with chicken or fish. This makes dining out easy.

## NuTricia's T Plan

I also recommend using my **NuTricia's T plan** for ordering. It helps you keep perspective on your eating as both a weekly and a daily process.

The T looks like this:

What Did I Eat the Rest of the Week?

What

Did

I

Eat

Today?

Look at how you ate across the week. Did you eat fried food this week? Yes, well, then it's not a good idea to order it tonight. Have I eaten at least two fish meals this week? No. Then, order some fish tonight. Then look down along the stem of the T, which represents what you ate today. Did you eat vegetables today? Not much. Okay, let's order a salad and make it a veggie-heavy meal. Did you eat red meat today? Yes, then don't order meatballs tonight. How about a bean-rich meal? Perhaps a bean soup and a salad?

Also, if you choose to indulge in an alcoholic drink, then forgo dessert. If you have a piece of bread, then don't eat the rice or pasta that comes with your meal. If you are trying to lose weight and eat all courses, including drink/s and dessert, then it will be hard to achieve your goal. However, if you plan a small indulgence and keep the rest of the meal healthy, you can stay on track.

## NuTricia's Takeaways

Since people seem busier than ever, picking up food on the run is often a quick meal solution. Unfortunately, this can come with some pitfalls, particularly if you're not careful. While you certainly can enjoy yourself and go out to dinner when you're watching your weight and/or trying to eat more healthfully, it's best to have a plan and make good choices!

**Here are some key points:**

- Choose quality over quantity.
- Ask for the veggie of the day.
- Pack up half to go.
- Save yourself grief — go online and look at the menu beforehand.
- Avoid saucy, cheesy, and fried foods.
- Remember, fried food doubles the calories.
- Have a go-to meal, such as a salad with chicken or fish.

# INVESTMENT:

## FITNESS AND WEIGHT MANAGEMENT

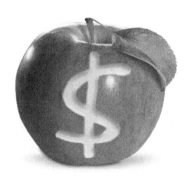

# CHAPTER 5

# Moving Your Body

Moving your body earns you a multitude of dividends, especially when balanced with good nutrition and healthy habits. I use this section to focus on movement, and the fantastic impact it can have on your health, your mood, your body, and your life. Adding in even a little movement into your life means you'll feel better, live longer, and lose or maintain your weight.

The best part is a secret that fitness enthusiasts have known for a long time: moving more is the fountain of youth. Over the past 20 years working in the health industry, I have seen this over and over again. While attending conferences, I've met numerous fitness professionals and enthusiasts who appear much younger than their ages. It's not only in their faces, but also in the youthful, smooth way their bodies move.

Moving your body can lead to success in other areas of your life as well. It can make you feel better overall, enhance your self-esteem, and prevent and treat burnout. After my second pregnancy, I was feeling sluggish and having a hard time bouncing back. I decided to get motivated by going to a personal trainer. After just one session, my legs felt so much stronger. Since then, I've had similar experiences where just one class helps me discover muscles I never knew I had. A particularly memorable class was with Speedball creator and boxing expert Steve Feinberg. I was challenged in class, and the next day felt the challenge in my muscles. It's amazing how just one movement class or session can have such a strong effect on how you feel physically and mentally.

> ## To learn more about Steve and his inspiring story, check out my free bonus chapter at:
>
> ## www.triciasilverman.com/book

## 10 Ways to Help You Invest in Moving Your Body

Movement is slowly being engineered out of our lives. Think about your car. Do you remember 30 years ago when the locks had to be pulled up and down? If you picked up a friend, you had to lean over the passenger seat to unlock the door. To pull up the window, you had to use your biceps to crank the handle around and around. What about turning your key? Some newer car models just require the push of a button. The way things are going, if we don't seek out purposeful physical activity, the only strong muscles we will have will be in our fingers.

I'm not saying we have to do away with all modern conveniences, but we do need to be thoughtful about making sure we move and challenge our bodies. Remember how I started the book by talking about how a healthy life is all about making small choices? This is it. Are you going to take the stairs or the escalator? I'm encouraging you to take the stairs on your journey to being physically fit. What's ahead are easy-to-follow steps to get you started on a successful movement journey.

# 1. Find your passion.

Finding your fitness passion may take some trial and error, and it may even change over time. But it's so exciting when you find one. I tend to go through phases of loving and enjoying one fitness format, then shifting to take on a different fitness challenge. The following are some of my fitness passions over the years: Zumba, belly dancing, Tai Chi, yoga, Beachbody programs, Jane Fonda videos, Richard Simmons videos, Tami Lee Webb's Buns of Steel, Tae Bo, exercise bands, barre classes, Hip Hop Abs, walking, biking, hiking, jogging, and more. If you don't try different fitness, movement, and dance formats, you'll never know where your passion lives. And, trying new classes and techniques can keep you motivated and inspired to keep moving. It's fun!

If you are bored with your current fitness choices or find it hard to get motivated, take baby steps to ease yourself into something new. For instance, if you want to try a gentle yoga class, then today or this week, investigate where gentle yoga classes are available near you. Tomorrow or next week, call to inquire about the costs or any other questions you may have. Then, commit to a date in the next two weeks when you'll attend a class. Breaking the steps down into smaller, more manageable tasks makes it easier to get started and to find your fitness passion.

Your passions can follow you or change throughout your life. One fond memory that I have is when I went ballroom dancing with my husband, his father, and his father's girlfriend. The ballroom was full of people of all ages. Couples in their 80s were dancing gracefully and were in amazing shape. I want that to be me in my 80s. How about you?

## Motivated by the Cheering Crowds

When I asked Doree if her 100 pound weight loss had led to success in her life, she zeroed in on the 5Ks, 10Ks, and half marathons she is able to run now as a result of transforming her body through good nutrition and exercise. For her, the exhilaration of running the race, hearing the crowds cheer, and getting a ribbon is a feeling like no other, and *a feeling she never knew was possible when she was sedentary and weighing in at over 230 pounds* for her 5'3" frame. Doree, a 59-year-old married mom of two, also mentioned that her weight loss had strengthened her family, a success factor in itself.

Losing weight also notably increased Doree's self-confidence and self-esteem. She now has the confidence to speak in front of people, when in the past, she would have shied away from presentations and public speaking. Doree's turning point and motivation for losing weight were related to her health. She was in her mid-40s and felt her weight was diminishing her health.

## Doree's Exercise Advice

"Try something different that works for you as an individual. Find something that makes you happy."

Doree also shared some interesting insights on both exercise and nutrition, "Getting in control is empowering." I couldn't agree with her statement more. I know personally when I am eating well and staying on track with my exercise, I feel an amazing inner source of strength.

Formerly, over 100 pounds ago, Doree's spare time activities included needlepoint, calligraphy, and reading. Now, physical activity is an important part of her spare time. Doree exercises most days. She does strength training three times per week. She runs every other day and takes spin classes. She also swims and enjoys cross-country skiing.

Doree has been able to maintain her weight loss. "It's been close to 10 years now that I have managed to keep the weight off through healthy eating and exercise. A big accomplishment for a former yo-yo dieter!"

Follow Doree at her Facebook page titled, Weight Loss with Doree: The Weight is Over: facebook.com/Weight-Loss-with-Doree-The-Weight-is-Over-165783320170740/

**Doree before:**                    **Doree after**

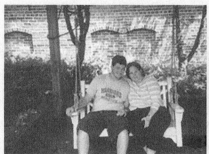 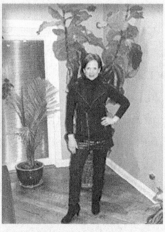

To find out more about organized walks for charity and races in your area, check out www.active.com.

## 2. Move More at Work.

Incorporating movement into your workday is a relatively straightforward change that can pay big dividends for your body and health. It's easy to lose track of time and find yourself hours later sitting in the same place, working on a task. The result may be a sore neck, achy back, or dry eyes.

To combat these symptoms, add in short bouts of physical activity. Again, it doesn't have to be much. A quick loop around the office can be enough to restart your body. Some fitness watches will even remind you to get up and move.

One of the best things that you can do for you and your employer is to walk during lunch and whenever else possible during the workday. Moving enhances creativity, is wonderful for your circulation, and can help you control your blood sugar levels. Even if you only have a few minutes to move, no worries. It's not all or nothing. Small bouts of movement count.

It's also a good idea to take eye breaks to avoid vision strain. Follow the 20-20-20 rule: Look away from the computer screen about every 20 minutes and look at something 20 feet away for 20 seconds.[40] Performing this small task can reduce eyestrain and improve vision.

Finally, don't eat and work (or use a computer or phone) at the same time. Take a break to enjoy your meal and possibly a nice conversation with someone else. Or take a fitness break. Many companies recognize the importance of their employees' health and wellness and have started to offer fitness classes during the day, so employees can take a break and do something they enjoy.

## 3. Practice the 7-Minute Workout.

Dr. Oz recommends that everyone, even the busiest people, start their day with a seven-minute workout. He's even created a variety of seven-minute workout videos with fitness trainers. When I first heard of this idea, it caught my attention and really stuck with me.

How about you? If you are really busy, can you find just seven minutes in the morning to do some type of movement? Maybe it's yoga, maybe strength exercises, maybe dancing. It can change your whole mindset for the day.

## 4. Multitask Your Exercise.

Sometimes it feels like there aren't enough hours in the day to get everything done and exercise. But there's no excuse not to move. On days when you feel like there's simply not enough time, you can multitask your exercise by pairing your movement with other tasks. It sounds a little crazy, but it's a technique I use all of the time. Basically I add a little extra movement to something I'm already doing.

Here are a few ways you can multitask your exercise:

1. Dance or march while doing dishes or folding laundry.
2. Have to pick up and clean around the house? Set a timer for 20-30 minutes, turn up the music and dance or march your way around the house.
3. Commit to something small! Spend just 5 to 10 minutes on the treadmill, stationary bike, elliptical, or other home exercise device and complete other tasks at the same time—opening mail, answering emails or texts, reading documents for work, etc. These short bouts add up throughout the day,

and just five to 10 minutes of movement can improve your mindset for the rest of the day.

4. Change your perspective on TV viewing. Only watch TV if you are moving at the same time. You can be on a treadmill, lifting weights, doing yoga, or doing body-weight strength moves.

## 5. See a Personal Trainer.

To really kickstart a workout program, find a personal trainer. It can be a game changer for your health and motivation! A good trainer works with you to identify your goals and then creates a fun, challenging workout that moves you forward. While one-on-one training sessions may cost a little more than classes, the results are phenomenal. You can also control costs by having one personal training session per week (or every two weeks) where you get a plan and then work out on your own. Or you can try small group personal training. Many gyms offer this. It's smaller than a group class, but the trainer is training more than one person. You pay less for this than you do for personal, one-on-one training, but get more individualized attention than in a group class.

What I love about personal trainers is that each one is unique. Just like finding the right doctor or psychologist, you may have to go through a few trainers to find the one who suits you best. While working out at the gym, I noticed one particular trainer, named Bern Prince, who was always loud — laughing, and having fun with his clients—while at the same time putting them through hardcore workouts. I decided this was the right personality fit for me and, boy, was I right.

You want to find a trainer whose personality suits you, and creates training sessions that challenge you. The personality and motivational abilities of your trainer are really important. And let me stress, everyone's personality is different. If you are serious and quiet, you will probably have a different trainer than me. There is no right or wrong to this. It's like finding the right way to lose weight. We are all unique.

For a good idea on how one of my favorite personal trainers thinks, check out the insights from Bern. He's now a Boston-based personal trainer and CrossFit instructor at Invictus Boston, an elite CrossFit gym.

He's one of the most fun, creative, and effective athletes I have ever trained with.

## Bern Prince on Spot Reduction

There are many different opinions on spot reduction of areas of the body that people would like to minimize through exercise. Bern gives us some hope. "You can definitely spot reduce. There would be no such thing as a bodybuilder if you couldn't spot reduce. It's hard, but yes, it can be done." Doesn't this make sense to you, as you picture bodybuilders in your mind?

## Bern on BS

Too tired to exercise? Bern says, "Stop BS-ing! If you want to make it a priority, you will find time." Don't you love Bern already?

## Bern on the Greatest Benefits of Exercise

"Exercise gives you confidence, improves your health, and boosts your energy levels. Confidence is impressive; it makes you attractive, intriguing, and intimidating. Most of America covers up, or wants to be covered. One important reason for exercising is to feel comfortable in your own skin."

## Bern on Success and Hiring a Personal Trainer

"Hiring a personal trainer can help you to get comfortable in your own skin and get more confidence. You can tell right away when someone doesn't have it, and is insecure. I've seen lawyers, CEOs, police officers, and others turn into 14-year-olds in the gym because they are not comfortable in their own skin." Personal trainers want to help you. They can help you attack and attain a goal because they offer you a path to success and accountability along the way. When you succeed, it leads to a fitter body and a more confident self.

Bern recalls one client who, during her first few sessions, was "turned off and grumpy." Before starting with Bern, she had worked with many trainers and not found the right fit. He shifted the dynamic by having an honest, open conversation with her about goals and how to achieve them. Through his training sessions and guidance, she lost 13 pounds in just two months! "She is noticeably happier."

Another client, who used to live on the StairMaster, started working with Bern and learned how to use other equipment in the gym. She started strength training, and doing more targeted exercises. Through his direction, she got ripped pretty fast. She can now deadlift 185 pounds (no small feat) and can do four sets of 10 pull-ups (this brings to mind Linda Hamilton's guns [well-sculpted arms] from *Terminator 2* in the 90s). He noticed that she is smiling more, and has more confidence in her presence and appearance.

## Bern on How Often to Work Out

Bern says, "At least 4 times a week. Your dentist would laugh if you said I brush my teeth three times per week."

---

### Bern's Personal Fitness Regimen

Bern practices what he preaches. He does resistance exercise six days a week for an hour and a half each day, working out different body parts each day. Three days a week, he does endurance exercise such as running or rowing with a specific distance in mind. One day a week is a recovery day with no formal exercise planned.

---

## 6. Find an Accountability Partner.

Accountability partners make sure you follow through with the goals you set. I think this is the secret to success—finding people who know what you want and are motivated to help you achieve it. Having a trainer to be accountable to is helpful, but others can be your accountability partners and fitness buddies as well. As a wellness and nutrition coach, I have been this person for many people, so I see the success that having a person to be accountable to can bring.

You can ask neighbors or family members to work out with you and hold you accountable. You can rely on the friends you walk with who expect you on the path at 6 a.m., no excuses. You can join fitness challenges on social media. At the gym, you can find like-minded people by joining classes and introducing yourself.

Having someone to be accountable to can help you stay motivated because it makes you feel that you are part of something bigger than yourself. Another person has a vested interest in your wellness achievements.

## 7. Find a Home Fitness Solution.

At-home workouts are a fantastic workout option, and there are countless possibilities available on DVDs and online. My first encounter with home fitness started when I saw a cool infomercial for the Beachbody fitness star, Shaun T., and his Hip Hop Abs program. I bought the DVD and loved it. His Beachbody programs, such as Insanity and Cize, have produced a loyal following who have transformed their bodies through his tutelage.

I was really psyched when I heard he would be speaking at a fitness conference organized by Kevin Lopes, a police officer from Massachusetts. You'll learn about Kevin's transformation shortly.

One of my clients recently raved about her favorite fitness DVD that featured fitness video icon Keli Roberts. How fortunate that I have gotten to meet the lovely and talented Keli Roberts at SCW Fitness Conferences. Check out Keli's videos at http://www.keliroberts.com/shop/.

Your local library is another source of fun fitness DVDs. I have found many great dance, yoga, and kettlebell workouts in the library's DVD section. Your cable service may also offer on-demand fitness options.

If you surf the internet and YouTube for fitness, be sure that the instructors teaching the classes you take are certified to teach. One of my favorite go-to places for workout ideas is Chris Freytag's Get Healthy U website: GetHealthyU.com/. Look around the site for helpful exercises, tough workouts, and wellness resources. If you're a fitness instructor looking for new ideas, then check out SCW On-Demand at https://scwfit.com/store/on-demand/. There are hundreds of fitness videos with instructor tips and demonstrations for a low monthly cost.

## 8. Get Outside and Build Movement into Your Lifestyle.

In Italy, after a meal, people enjoy a Passeggiata, also known as an enjoyable stroll. If we change our mindset and think of taking an enjoyable stroll after dinner, rather than exercising, it may be more apt to happen. Getting out in nature can make you feel really good. Have you hiked on a trail lately? There is something to be said for connecting with nature, and the effect it has on your mental state. Research from the UK has found that walking in nature can put you in a meditative state.[41] Gardening, raking leaves, shoveling snow, skiing, swimming, and biking all get you outside. I find bike riding on bike trails particularly enjoyable.

When my family goes on trips, we look for hiking, biking, and walking opportunities. What about the rest of the year? Can you walk to or from a train station that is one stop further than where you need to get on or off? Can you do stair walking, or walk through your building during lunch? Can you walk or bike to work, or to do errands? I like to use CVS, or the library as a destination for a walk. There's always something you need at CVS, and the library is one of my favorite places.

So, pick a destination for your walk and get going. You can also pick a theme for your walk. When we were renovating my house, I would walk or bike with the theme of looking at everyone's front door for color and style ideas. I did the same thing with outside lanterns. You wouldn't believe how many different lanterns there are out there! Go ahead and make this a theme! Also, consider planning walking excursions with friends, rather than meeting up for food.

Once you've started a fitness program, you're going to be surprised at how easily you can make it a part of your life. You'll find you enjoy it and won't want to miss a workout. That means you need to schedule your workouts like you do any important commitment. Once you have these times on your calendar, they become what you do, and you're less likely to miss them. And if you start to slip, your accountability partners can help you stay on track.

Additionally, by following a regular exercise program, you'll find you have more energy and confidence, and generally feel better about yourself. You'll want to be more active the rest of your day by taking walks, bike rides, etc.

## Join the SWAT Team!

Yes, that's right! Another benefit of exercise is that you can get yourself in such good shape that you can make the SWAT team. Remember Kevin Lopes? That's exactly what he did! Of course, you have to be a police officer first.

Kevin was in the Army National Guard during college. After 9/11, he served as a military police officer and later became a civilian police officer. After four years of working late nights, going through a bad divorce, and having a stressful job and home life, Kevin had gained over 40 pounds. He battled his weight at the gym but didn't see the results he was looking for. He wanted a program that would help him return to his military shape and endurance.

Kevin's brother had recently lost weight and was in great shape from doing Beachbody's P90X DVD program developed by Tony Horton. One day, he convinced Kevin to try it with him.

Kevin's first P90X workout was plyometrics, and he was hooked. "I hadn't had a workout like that in years! It felt great to sweat." He began to do the P90X program regularly.

Kevin lost about 30 pounds, and people started to talk. "Many guys at work asked me what I did to lose all my weight, and I told them P90X! It was great to be able to answer, just like my brother did for me."

After finishing the 90-day P90X program, Kevin pushed his body even further and started the Beachbody Insanity program. He lost an additional 10 pounds, but more importantly, he was now in the best shape of his life. He felt in better shape than while serving his country in the military.

Kevin lost 40 pounds in 120 days through the Beachbody programs! He went from 210 to 170 pounds, while building muscle mass. He was in better shape than in high school!

For Kevin, the beauty of transforming into a leaner cut physique was only the beginning of his success streak. Kevin had long aspired to be a member of the Fall River Police Department's elite SWAT Team, or Emergency Services Unit, as it is now known. Acceptance to this unit involves a careful review of an applicant's job performance, awards, and certificates, as well as a successfully completing a tough physical fitness test.

Kevin stood out from his competitors on the physical fitness test. The group had to race up 14 flights of stairs and then back down 14, which Kevin accomplished in 10 minutes and 30 seconds. He beat the other contenders in the running race section by three minutes. The group then had to do one minute of push-ups. He told the others taking the test that he would do 80 push-ups—a lofty goal that no one believed. Then, he not only did 80 but also "10 more for each one of them taking the test."

Kevin made the SWAT team! He would never have been able to do this during his first five years as a police officer. I always knew the SWAT team was an elite group of police officers, but I never knew much more about this amazing group. When I asked Kevin to explain what the SWAT team is, he explained, "The SWAT team? They're who the police go to when they have a 911 emergency." Pretty awesome, huh? "Being in the best shape is critical as a member of the SWAT team in case I have to chase someone or run away."

Because of Kevin, I was able to meet Shaun T., the elite fitness trainer from the Beachbody Insanity workout series. Kevin arranged and sponsored a conference starring Shaun T. at the famous Gillette Stadium in Foxborough, Massachusetts.

## 9. Follow Inspirational Fitness Experts on Social Media and in Print.

Get inspired! Follow fitness trendsetters on Instagram and Facebook. In addition to workout tips, they never fail to motivate and encourage you to be the best you.

I have been blessed to be a part of the SCW Fitness Educational Company's National Conferences. Check out the MANIA® Fitness conferences here: SCWFit.com/Mania/. Click on the next national conference that is coming up and then click on presenters. If you start following me on Facebook, you'll see that I follow MANIA® presenters. They have helped my own fitness regimen and the classes I teach improve by leaps and bounds.

The following fitness experts are always sharing fun, effective moves to help you get or stay fit.

Abbie Appel on Instagram: https://www.instagram.com/abbieappel/
Chris Freytag on Facebook: Facebook.com/chrisfreytagpage/
Yury Rockit on Instagram: https://www.instagram.com/yuryrockit/

When purchasing fitness books, be sure that the instructors have fitness certifications. One book that I often recommend to clients is *A Women's Guide to Muscle and Strength* by Irene Lewis-McCormick.

## 10. Follow Current Physical Fitness Guidelines and Train Your Body to Last a Long Time.

Current U.S. fitness guidelines recommend that individuals get 150 to 300 minutes (or two hours 30 minutes to five hours) of moderate intensity exercise, or 75 to 150 minutes (one hour 15 minutes to two hours 30 minutes) of vigorous exercise per week.[42] For even greater health benefits, aim to go beyond 300 minutes of moderate intensity exercise or 150 minutes of vigorous intensity exercise each week. You can also combine moderate and vigorous exercise. Moderate exercise is what's often referred to as "cardio." Examples of cardio include walking briskly, biking, swimming, raking leaves, and other activities that raise your heart rate. Vigorous cardio includes jogging, running, or shoveling snow.

Past guidelines recommended getting your minutes of exercise in at least 10-minute increments, but the new guidelines say that it doesn't have to be in 10-minute segments. So, the takeaway here is to move when you can! One of the things I have been using for some of my clients is a minutes per week goal to help them meet these requirements. We break down where and when they are going to get their 150 to 300+ minutes of cardio. You might want to consider this to help you meet the guidelines. And then enjoy the wellness dividends!

The guidelines also state that, "Adults should also do muscle-strengthening activities of moderate or greater intensity and that involve all major muscle groups on 2 or more days a week, as these activities provide additional health benefits."[43] The major muscle groups are the legs, hips, chest, back, abdomen, shoulders, and arms.

Balance training should be added for older adults. These individuals should incorporate as much movement into their day as their conditions and fitness levels allow.

If you have pain or disability in a certain area of your body, try to find ways to move other parts of your body. Seeing a physical therapist can help you to do this. They may also be able to help you strengthen your areas of weakness, potentially eliminating or diminishing your pain issues. I found it fascinating to learn that by strengthening weaknesses in my hips and feet, I was able to solve the pain I was having in my ankle.

I also was fascinated when I learned the following from fitness icon Lawrence Biscontini regarding how strengthening the front of my lower legs can help prevent me from shuffling as I get older: Lawrence shared that, "One of the recent developments in research in gait efficiency discusses the role of our anterior tibialis to help dorsiflex our ankles [by pulling up your toes] to avoid shuffling and to help clear obstacles when our toes catch on objects or we start to trip. To be sure, stability and mobility training (muscular endurance, strength, and flexibility) for all major muscle groups proves necessary with active aging, but this long-overlooked muscle group is a recently-discovered potential life-saver when trained regularly."

## Preventing the Shuffle

Help stop and prevent shuffling feet with this shin-strengthening exercise:

While sitting in a chair with your feet on the floor, lift your toes and the front of your feet toward your shins (keeping your heels on the ground), and hold for one to two seconds. Return to starting position. Aim for eight to 15 repetitions. Do one to two sets on two to three non-consecutive days per week. In a few weeks, you can progress to doing this exercise while standing, holding onto something for balance. This exercise helps to strengthen the tibialis anterior, which is a muscle that runs from your foot to the upper part of your tibia. To keep your body balanced, it's also good to strengthen the opposing muscles, which are the calf muscles, gastrocnemius, and soleus. A physical therapist or personal trainer are the best sources for ideas for strengthening specific muscle groups, so your body functions optimally.

Many group fitness instructors and personal trainers are now incorporating more functional fitness moves into their programs. Functional fitness exercises often use more than one joint and muscle at a time, and help to strengthen your body for the activities that you do in daily living. It moves beyond sitting at a machine at the gym and working one body part at a time. Examples are squats, lunges, and the way your body moves in a yoga or Tai Chi class.

Remember to check with your doctor before beginning a new fitness regime.

## NuTricia's Takeaways

Investing in moving your body will lead to numerous healthy dividends, such as feeling great, losing weight, living longer, and more. The key is to find movement that you enjoy. Here are some key takeaways from this chapter:

- Move when you can, even if you only have a few minutes. Some exercise is better than none.
- Multitask your exercise—bike to work, dance while doing dishes, etc.
- Plan movement into your calendar.
- Aim to work up to at least 150 minutes per week of moderate intensity cardio or 75 minutes of vigorous cardio.
- Do exercises to strengthen major muscle groups at least twice per week.
- See a physical therapist to help relieve pain.

---

CHAPTER 6

# Smart Weight Loss

## Success Factors for Weight Loss

Smart weight loss strategies that work for you are your success factors. In this chapter, I've collected the strategies my clients have found most successful for them. This is not an all or nothing approach. You need to identify the changes and habits that work for you, so I suggest you just try some of the ideas listed. See what works for you and what doesn't.

When you're having success, it's easier to stick to your wellness plan. If your weight starts creeping up, make sure you implement your success factors. Investing in effective weight loss strategies results in amazing dividends: such as feeling better, losing or maintaining weight, and feeling more in control.

My clients have done so well with finding and using these success factors! I wish the same for you!

### Success Factor #1 – Avoid or Limit Trigger Foods

Are your trigger foods holding you back from weight loss? Do you know your trigger foods? They are different for everyone. Mine are dry cereal, crackers, candy, and other sugary treats. When I start eating these, it's often hard to stop which can get in the way of my weight management goals.

Chocolate is a huge trigger for many people. One client would come home from work and eat a popular chocolate candy. Once she had her chocolate fix, she started craving another fix ... can you guess which type? Salt! She would drive to fast-food restaurants to satisfy her salt craving. Once we got her off the chocolate candy, she no longer craved the salty food.

What about you? Are there certain trigger foods that lead you down a slippery slope? Perhaps they are even healthy foods, like peanut butter. Consider drawing up a list of your trigger foods and commit to staying away from these foods while you are trying to lose weight. Or, if it's easier, give yourself a specific time frame (one or two weeks to start) when you won't eat your trigger foods. See how you feel and how it impacts your weight. Perhaps once you feel more in control, you can start adding these foods back in with portion-sized amounts.

One thing to remember is that some of these trigger foods, like sugar, are highly addictive and light up the brain, igniting our reward center, so we want more. The combination of salt, sugar, and fat can be particularly tricky for many of us. Think about restaurant food, and the appetizers and meals and desserts. These foods create memories when we eat them, so we keep seeking them out, and return to the restaurant to get another fix. The best bet is to limit trying new sugary, salty, fat-rich, ultra-indulgent foods.

## Success Factor #2 – Eat More Mindfully

"Do we eat too much?" Horace Fletcher posed this question over 100 years ago and answered it by saying that nine out of ten doctors say "Yes." We're still eating too much and even more than in the early

1900s. However, the wisdom of Horace Fletcher may help you to enjoy your food a bit more. In his book *The A.B. - Z of Our Own Nutrition*, he stated that "Proper mastication and insalivation (mixing with saliva), give your sense of taste far greater gastronomic enjoyment than you have ever before had."[44] He called this "economic nutrition," but we call it mindful eating. As you chew your food more, you slow down the rate and amount you eat.

Mindful eating is one of the best practices you can learn to help control your eating. I think the practice of yoga supports mindful eating. A lovely participant in one of my nutrition series classes came in laughing one week. When I asked what was so funny, he told me that through mindful eating for one week he had lost four pounds. The habit he focused on was not watching the television while he ate. A recent study on women in Ghana found that increased television watching is associated with overweight and obesity.[45]

Over 16 years, ago mindless eating grew on me, literally. I had developed what looked like a tire of fat, right around my middle. I was letting stress get the best of me and had started using food to stuff down my feelings and disappointments. I had moved, gotten married, and started a new job, all within a couple of months. The stress was too much, and I was anesthetizing myself with food. One of the primary culprits was a trigger food I mentioned earlier—dry cereal. And it was a healthy brand of dry cereal. But it didn't matter that it was "healthy." You can gain weight eating healthy food, too. Quantity matters. I ate too much of it every day after work, repeating what I did years earlier in high school when I came home from school and ate endless bowls of cereal while watching soap operas. Once I started eating mindfully and not drowning my sorrows with food, the weight came off, in both instances.

Mindful eating is a conscious effort to slow down the rate at which you eat, to chew your food more, to tune in to the experience, and to savor every bite.

## A Mindful Approach Led to a 100-Pound Weight Loss

Carrie Verrocchio is an inspirational life coach who lost over 100 pounds using a mindful approach. I met Carrie when she attended my nutrition session at an SCW Fitness Conference. She radiates positive energy and enthusiasm! She accomplished her weight loss by making small changes, such as eating more vegetables, drinking more water, looking at recipes and ingredients, and cutting out refined foods.

Carrie listens to her body to notice if she is hungry. If she's not hungry, she doesn't eat. She also doesn't obsess ... she lets her body tell her what it needs. She uses prayer and meditation, as well. Also, the faith-based book, *Thin Within* by Judy Halliday helped shape some of her philosophies around eating.[46] One of Carrie's philosophies involves not watching too much television because it is a trigger for her to eat. However, one of the things that she did find helpful on television was an infomercial for Beachbody, a popular fitness platform, which offers fitness videos and coaching.

Carrie now has certification in five Beachbody formats and teaches live every Saturday. Carrie shared, "This gives me a way to reach out, to help people to not be afraid to move, no matter what their age or weight. This gives me an outlet to be compassionate because I've been there. I love it!" Carrie has maintained her weight loss for 15 years.

These are Carrie's before and after pics. People that know me from my childhood may think the before pic is me. Carrie and I may be long-lost twins!!

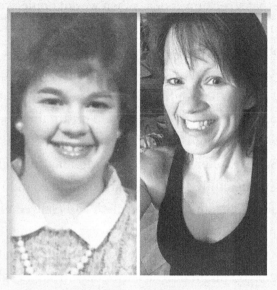

## Success Factor #3 – Time Your Meals

Aim to eat your largest meal at lunch and eat it before 3 p.m. Researchers have found that people who did this tended to lose more weight when compared with people who ate their main meal after 3 p.m.[47]

I also suggest avoiding getting overly hungry and maintaining maximum energy levels by eating roughly every three to four hours.

## Success Factor #4 – Avoid "Freakend" Eating

When I was a kid, my family would do family "pigouts." Yes, that's what we called them. We would go with my father to his deli on Saturday nights. While he closed the deli and did the accounting for the week, we would roam the store, gathering food for the pigout that was to take place somewhere around 11 p.m. when we returned home. While we picked food for the pigout, I would eat ice cream sandwiches and anything else that struck my fancy. When we got home, we would scarf down Entenmann's chocolate chip cookies, Hershey's chocolate chip ice cream, potato chips, and whatever else we had picked out.

On Sunday morning, my dad would get up early to open the deli, and around 9 or 10 a.m., would return home with a huge bag of bagels plus other treats, like crumb cake, Boston cream donuts, scones, and half-moon cookies. I would eat some of these sugary treats, plus several bagels on a Sunday, often losing count. Monday through Friday, we would eat pretty healthily, so it was hard to understand why I was an overweight kid. As an adult, I did the math and realized for me as a kid (and for so many kids and adults), the weekend eating was wreaking havoc on my weight. It's very easy on a Saturday and Sunday to gain back any weight you might have lost Monday through Friday. I call this "freakend" eating.

I've noticed that way too many people eat pretty darn well Monday through Friday afternoon. They would earn an A or A+ if they were to be graded. This is often followed by unstructured eating that starts with Friday drinks and restaurant meals and continues until Sunday, probably earning them an F. I'd rather they be a B or B+ student every day, having consistency with their healthy eating that weaves its way through the entire week. Some small indulgences can be planned in, but a "cheat day" or complete "freakend" will likely cause you to gain back any weight you've lost Monday through Friday. I've done the math. Only one day of "freakend" eating can undermine five to six days of healthful eating when it comes to results on the scale.

## Success Factor #5 – Embrace Salads and Vegetables

The sooner you embrace vegetables, the easier losing weight will be and the longer your life will be. An attendee of one of my wellness programs shared with me that he had lost over 100 pounds through a program at his gym. One of the success factors that helped him with his weight loss was switching from sandwiches to salads for lunch. Another attendee at one of my employee wellness programs, manages his weight by eating what he calls "garbage pail lunches," instead of sandwiches. The lunches are leftovers from home-cooked vegetarian dinners that he dumps over salad greens. Read more about his story here: https://www.triciasilverman.com/nutrition.

Another tactic is to eat a salad before your meals, which can help you take in fewer calories for the entire meal.[48] Fruit can do the same thing. Apples, in particular, are very filling and have been shown to enhance satiety.

## Success Factor #6 – Use Food Tracking Apps

I find it interesting when diet books and articles say that weight loss is not about the calories, yet when you take a closer look, their suggested meal plans **are** about the calories. Losing weight is simply about eating less and moving your body. The hard part is figuring how to do this in a way that allows you to be a happy, thriving human at the same time!

One suggestion I make to clients that works like a charm is to use a food tracking app. These apps can help you because they give you a budget of calories, or you set your own budget, and then you track the foods you eat so you don't go over your budget. The apps force you to look at portion size, which is so critical to losing weight. When using the apps, notice how larger portion sizes equal more calories. It can be quite eye-opening.

These apps are your friends, and they are free. You can get added functionality by paying a little bit more, and in some cases, it may be worth it, depending on how detailed you want to be. A few that my clients have used include LoseIt, MyFitnessPal, and Sparkpeople. The LoseIt app is very user-friendly and has nice, colorful icons that make it fun to use! MyFitnessPal is very popular, especially among personal trainers and fitness enthusiasts, because it allows you to track water intake and exercise.

Sparkpeople is another great app and has a large community that shares recipes and offers helpful blogs and articles. (My quick mason jar soup article, as well as various quotes from me, appears in the helpful community section of their website.)

Which is the best app? It's the one your friends, family, or co-workers are using. Why? Because you can ask them to show you how to use it. They can answer questions, and cut the learning curve for you.

## Success Factor #7 – Create a Meal Plan

Creating a meal plan involves setting a schedule that tells you what food or food groups you're going to eat and when. It takes the uncertainty out of mealtime because you already decided on what to eat for a healthy lunch or dinner. I put a sample 1,600 calorie meal plan in the appendix B. I find that very detailed-oriented people do well with meal plans. A registered dietitian is the best suited professional for creating a meal plan.

## Finding and Optimizing Your BMR

BMR stands for Basal Metabolic Rate. Basically, it tells you the number of calories you need for your body to perform daily functions. Apps often underestimate your nutrition needs. In fact, dietitians often use two formulas to determine your specific calorie needs—both the Mifflin St. Jeor and Harris-Benedict.

To save you time from doing lengthy calculations, go to BMRCalculator.org, and you will get your calorie needs for weight maintenance. Don't forget to scroll down to see the numbers listed in the charts that also take into account activity level. Once you figure out your maintenance calories, you subtract 500 to lose a pound a week, or 250 to lose half a pound a week. Since no calculation is perfect and our bodies are all unique, it's a good idea to experiment with calorie budgets to find the budget for you that gives you weight loss without being hungry.

So, let's say that you are a 50-year-old, 5' 4", 155-pound female. The Mifflin St. Jeor calculation on BMRCalculator.org shows that to maintain your weight at your current activity level of working out moderately three to five days per week, you'll need 2,033 calories per day (The Harris Benedict Equation estimates slightly higher at 2161 calories ... it's all an educated guess anyway, so pick one equation, or average the results of both equations, and go with it.). To lose a pound per week, you would need to eat 1,533 a day (2033 minus 500 calories). If your activity level increases, according to the chart on the website, to maintain your weight you'll need 2,262 calories a day, and to lose a pound a week, you'll need 1,762 calories a day.

Set your calorie budget on the fitness app somewhere in between the two numbers (the 1533 and the 1762) — say 1,600 calories — and eat up to this much each day for one to two weeks. See how your weight is impacted. Are you still hungry at this calorie level? Yes? Then increase your calories to 1,700 and after a week or so of eating 1,700 calories each day, notice the impact it had on your weight.

Consider yourself a science experiment. Another way you might want to use the app is to use it two days per week. This often keeps people on track, because they see how much food they need to eat in a day to lose weight, and it often carries over to other days. I have clients that use this strategy very successfully!

## Success Factor #8 – Use Smaller Plates and Have Multiple Measuring Cups and Spoons to Help You with Portion Sizes

These are the tools of the weight management trade. Smaller portions are essential for weight loss, and it helps to be able to measure and verify amounts before serving. I recommend having several sets of measuring cups and spoons in your kitchen, so you can determine portion size before putting food on a plate. And you'll always have another measuring spoon if one gets dirty.

Which bring us to the next step—plate size matters. In my *Sneaky Strategies to Manage Weight* presentation, I show participants how the same serving of rice looks bigger on a smaller plate. With smaller plates, you eat less, even though it may look like you are eating more! Guess what? Those eight large plates in your cabinet are now platters! Eat all meals off the smaller "lunch plate."

If plates matter, then so do utensils. Have you seen the size of the spoon that is given when you order gelato? I give out a similar spoon, also known as the #Silvermanspoon at some of my presentations. It encourages smaller bites and makes small indulgences last longer.

## Success Factor #9 – Get Food Off of Your Counters

When shopping for one of my past homes, I noticed there were always beautiful baked treats on the counter in eye-catching glassware, a wonderful invitation to eat too much sugar, get fat, and buy the house. I did one of the three! What I found interesting was that in another room, there were all these magazines on dieting. It's hard to diet when tasty treats are greeting you as you walk in the door.

A helpful weight loss secret is to sweep tempting food off your counters and get it into your cabinets. Another advantageous strategy when organizing your kitchen is to put healthy food in the refrigerator, so it's visible when you open the door. If you open your refrigerator after a long day of work and see fruit salad in a clear bowl, you're more likely to eat this. If you see pizza, you are more likely to eat that.

How you set up your cabinets is important, too. Put healthier items where you can see them and hide unhealthier items. Or better yet, don't keep them in your home. This is a great strategy for your trigger foods or foods like ice cream and cookies. I'm not saying never have them. Just don't keep them in the home. When you do want to indulge, don't waste time on junky stuff. Find the best quality homemade ice cream shop, or get a cookie from a bakery or a farmer's market. Why get store-bought treats that have all the junky ingredients? Don't waste your time, palate, and digestive system on #Industrialfood.

## Success Factor #10 – Get Support

Find a partner who brings expertise and can provide accountability. Having the support of a registered dietitian, wellness coach, and/or personal trainer can make a huge difference in your weight loss journey. This is a path that starts with you, but benefits from the support of others. You don't have to go it alone. In fact, there are also some weight loss programs and support groups that can be very helpful.

It's important to explore which programs have worked for you in the past. This is a learning opportunity. If you liked a program and lost weight while doing it in the past, let's figure out what worked, what didn't work, and what changes you might want to make. How can you approach that program differently this time, so you get lasting results?

Some programs that may be helpful:

- **Weight Watchers (WW)**
  Many people have been helped by WW meetings and the WW way of tracking food. I do suggest you read the labels carefully if considering any of their food products.

- **Overeater's Anonymous**
  This group helps people with issues around overeating, binge eating, over-exercising, and eating disorders. What I love about Overeater's Anonymous is that they have phone meetings most hours of the day throughout the week. You never have to be alone with your food issues since help is only a phone call away. They also have meetings where you can meet others face-to-face all over the country.

- **Food Addicts in Recovery Anonymous**
  This group helps people who are having issues as a result of their relationship with food and eating. I met an amazing, thin, beautiful woman who recently confided in me that this

group has changed her life and others as well. If you suspect you are a food addict, check out their website and their listing of meetings across the world: FoodAddicts.org.

## Losing Weight Impacted This Relationship Coach

"Being in better shape is going to help you in the dating world," says Adam LoDolce, world-renowned relationship expert and author of *Being Alone Sucks*. "You will see a much more attractive person in the mirror, which will raise your self-esteem, making you more attractive to other people."

LoDolce trimmed down to a sleek 185 pounds from a high of 230 pounds by joining Weight Watcher's (WW). "I decided to lose weight to feel better about myself. Essentially, I wanted to improve my self-image. My weight loss gave me more energy, self-confidence, and social freedom, the ability to say, feel, and act like your true self in any social situation, without fear of rejection or failure." Check out his website at SexyConfidence.com/ to learn more about Adam and the fascinating work he does as a motivational speaker and dating coach.

### Adam Before    Adam After

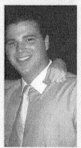 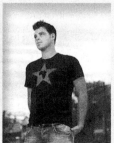

# Are You Addicted to Food?

Michael Prager has lost more than 600 pounds altogether, a result of losing and gaining weight until he finally lost the 155 pounds that has successfully kept him around 200 pounds for almost 30 years. Michael considers himself a food addict, and through therapy and support groups, he has been able to live a healthier, happier, and thinner life.

According to Michael, "People who are significantly overweight are not convinced they have a serious problem, partly because society doesn't think obesity has any causes more serious than laziness and personal failing." He found his food addiction to be a more serious problem that required more serious remedies.

Michael has revealed his fascinating story of addiction and recovery in *Fat Boy Thin Man*, which is available at his website, FatBoyThinMan.com. No longer a binge eater, Michael weighs and measures his food most days to help keep him on track. He avoids flour and refined sugar. "I am convinced my life is better off abstaining from these foods."

Some of the starchy food he enjoys includes beans, parsnips, potatoes, and whole grains, such as brown rice. "There's plenty of variety in my diet, no deprivation." Michael uses a food plan that was developed by a registered dietitian to guide his healthful way of eating. His mood and energy levels have been boosted by consistently eating based on his food plan and avoiding binge eating. In Michael's words, these strategies "have evened my temperament."

## Conquer Addictions, Enjoy Success

Michael's addictions to substances, including food, prevented him from enjoying meaningful romantic relationships in his 20s and early 30s. "Several factors made me unattractive, one was physical. I also embodied arrogance, self-centeredness, lack of honesty, and intimacy, among others. There were changes in my personality due to the treatment I got for food addiction. By conquering my food addiction, I was able to have my first girlfriend at 36 years old."

In the midst of his food addiction, Michael was demoted from his newspaper editing job because "I was childish and unable to get along with people." The same changes that led Michael to his romantic success also enabled him to achieve professional success at a higher career level. He was asked to be the editor of a section of a large newspaper. Currently, Michael is writing fiction, while also caring for the home for his family of three.

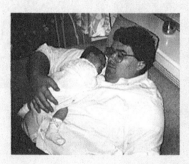 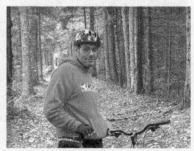

Food addiction exists, and it can really torment those who have it. The key is to get help. See a social worker or psychologist who has experience in this area and give the support groups mentioned previously a try.

## Success Factor # 11 – Practice Consistency to See Results

No matter what you decide to do about your weight and/or health, consistency is key. Roger Wright lost over 100 pounds in a year by committing to his personal trainer's requirement of "no excuses." He consistently watched what he ate and moved his body through running, swimming, cycling, and strength training. He's kept this weight off for over 10 years. Check out his transformation here: rfme.wordpress.com /f-or-videos/ Have you been consistent with your nutrition, fitness, and wellness endeavors? This can make the difference you are seeking.

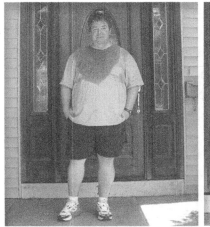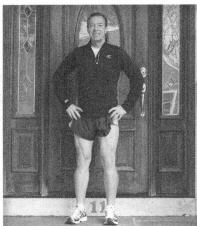

*Roger Before and After His Weight Loss*

## Success Factor # 12 – Rethink Your Drink

In one of my employee wellness programs, an attendee lost four pounds in one week from limiting how much beer she drank. At another program, I asked a participant to bring in the liquor glass he was drinking from because we were trying to guestimate how many calories he was taking in. He was shocked to discover he was drinking several hundred calories a day in alcohol. He immediately started curtailing his alcohol and made some positive nutrition changes, such as making new healthy recipes each week. He lost over 15 pounds in seven weeks.

The U.S. Dietary Guidelines state that women should limit alcoholic drinks to a maximum of one per day, and men should limit their drinks to a maximum of two per day. An alcoholic drink is defined as a 5-ounce glass of wine, a 12-ounce beer, or 1.5-ounces of 40% (80-proof) distilled spirits or liquor. However, even these amounts may be too much, especially if you're trying to lose weight.

### U.S. Standard Alcoholic Drink Portions

*Source: Centers for Disease Control and Prevention (CDC.*
*gov/Alcohol/Fact-Sheets/Moderate-Drinking.htm)*

I've discovered another interesting phenomenon; I like to call it the "wine belly." You may have seen a beer belly, and yes, this is a close cousin! More than one slender, 50-something woman has shown me the wine belly. They probably didn't think I would believe them since they looked fantastic. So, I've been flashed the wine belly. It is a belly that is easily covered up with clothes or a zip-up hoodie jacket, but to those who have it, it can be quite frustrating. The trend that leads to the wine belly occurs when a person gradually adds more wine to their diet until they notice they have a belly. They then seek the advice of a nutritionist, worried about this weight gain in the belly. The wine belly exists. Don't get me wrong … there's a sugar belly, too. But the wine belly exists and can be diminished by decreasing alcohol.

### Dietisms of the Pied Pipess

Remember Elizabeth? She's the dynamo who lost weight, and as a result, lost pain and didn't have to take numerous medications. Here are some of her diet tips, which I have coined "Dietisms."

- When beginning to lose weight, there is a period that is almost manic in nature, where everything is going well, and you are in the right frame of mind for losing weight. This period will end, and that is when you want to start making a promise to do one thing for the next week to make yourself healthier and to take better care of yourself. This is where Elizabeth's weekly classes really help because people are making promises to the group. You can make a promise to yourself, a registered dietitian, a journal, a personal trainer, a wellness coach, a supportive friend, or a support group, whatever works best for you.

- You need chocolate occasionally. Fit it in. Emotionally, sometimes you need candy. That's how to keep the weight off. The success of maintenance is at stake. You only want to lose weight once. When Elizabeth eats a small amount of candy, she realizes that "nothing bad happened," and she moves beyond it.

- In terms of reaching your goals, "take baby steps." "Even the snail reached the ark." (*I smile and think of a cute little snail inching his way toward the ark every time I read this saying! It makes so much sense to me! Thank you, Elizabeth!*)

To get more great tips from Elizabeth as well as helpful video snippets and smart "dietisms," check out her Facebook page — Losing Weight with Elizabeth: https://www.facebook.com/losing-weight-with-elizabeth-473204615724/. If you live in Connecticut, you can join Elizabeth's classes. For added inspiration, her books can be purchased on Amazon: *Born to be Fat* and *Losing Weight with Elizabeth*.

## Success Factor # 13 – Clobber Your Clutter

How messy is your home? Hoarding is associated with a higher BMI (body mass index — basically a higher weight per height) and binge-eating.[49] While you may not be a hoarder, it's much easier to make room for your wellness when you literally make room in your house for healthful activities. I have seen some of my coaching clients transform into healthier, happier, slimmer selves when they started to make time in their schedule to declutter.

Have you been putting off exercise in your home because there is nowhere to do it? You're not alone. Plan time in your calendar this week to start the decluttering process. Books that I've found helpful for decluttering:

- *The Life-Changing Magic of Tidying Up* by Marie Kondo
- *Lose the Clutter, Lose the Weight* by Peter Walsh

## Success Factor #14 – Minimize Dining Out, Maximize Healthy Choices When You Do

Restaurants represent a witch's brew of future health challenges, including outrageous portion sizes, hidden amounts of sugar, and unhealthy or poor quality ingredients. The amount of sugar in the specialty coffees at a popular donut shop is actually reckless. One of the best investments in your health that you can make is dining out less, and preparing more of your own meals and snacks. For details on how to make good choices when you do eat outside of the home, check out Chapter 4.

## Success Factor #15 – Develop Healthy Habits Beyond Food and Fitness

The success factors outlined above detail the most effective and practical weight loss strategies I've found. The final success strategy focuses on another essential aspect of wellness—healthy habits. These are the choices you make beyond nutrition and fitness that define how you live and thrive, including sleep, stress management, and staying connected to others. The next section provides more information on these healthy habits.

## NuTricia's Takeaways

Finding your success factors is one of the best things you can do for your wellness. Consider yourself a science experiment and try the suggested success factors in this chapter. See which ones work best for you, and use them whenever you might fall off track with your weight loss and wellness efforts. Here are some key takeaways:

- Keep your portion sizes small.
- Find someone to be accountable to.
- Choose one or two healthy habit changes or success factors to practice over the next week.
- Choose a food logging app or a meal plan to follow for weight loss.
- Limit your alcohol and dining out at restaurants.

# INVESTMENT:

## HEALTHY HABITS

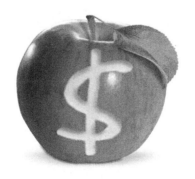

# CHAPTER 7

# Rev Your Engine for Energy and Productivity

The third investment we need to make for overall health and wellness involves lifestyle. To live well, you want to have the energy to do all that you'd like to do. We've talked about the importance of nutrition, but there are other strategies (beyond just choosing healthy foods) that you can employ to ensure you have the energy to be as productive as you possibly can be.

I learned this aspect of wellness the hard way during my dietetic internship. I would drink lots of caffeinated tea in the morning and during the day to "stay energized," then I would be wired at night and unable to sleep. I would take an over-the-counter sleep aid, and eventually get a few hours of restless sleep, just to repeat the pattern over again. And this lasted for months.

Toward the end of my internship, I planned a vacation for the one week I had between the end of my internship and the start of my first "real" job. My friends were all busy with their careers, so I decided to book a trip on my own to a health spa after seeing a postage stamp-sized advertisement for the Regency House Spa in Florida. This was back when the internet was pretty new, and you essentially could only search for your horoscope and the weather. So, I booked the entire trip based on this tiny ad and a quick call to the spa.

The picture in the ad showed a beautiful pool with a beautiful patio, overlooking the ocean. I thought, "There's no way it's going to look like that for the reasonable price I'm paying as a poor student." Oh boy, was I wrong. Not only was it as beautiful as the picture, but that week gave me insights that I value and cherish to this day.

Upon arrival, I discovered that the spa served vegan, no salt, no caffeine, and no alcohol meals. I was up for the challenge. After a few days of no caffeine (and a minor headache), I started to sleep like a baby. This was so eye-opening to me. I was able to stay off the sleep aid I'd been relying on. I slept soundly and had more energy during the day. I realized then that I am sensitive to caffeine, and now I rarely have it since it affects my sleep. In my classes, I've had several participants share their successes with going caffeine-free. Most report that they sleep better, think better, and feel more energized as a result.

An added benefit of the health spa visit was that I got to see how a truly healthy diet can impact not only how you feel, but also how you look (especially your skin). And I learned that just one week could have a measurable effect. I noticed at the end of the week that the other guests looked amazing and also seemed to feel great. They were less bloated, their skin was more radiant, and they appeared markedly happier.

## Eat for Energy

Even beyond the spa, a healthy diet can work wonders. One important way to eat more healthily involves having an eating plan. Instead of eating because it's a particular time of day, I recommend being proactive about meals—plan and decide not only what to eat, but also when the best time is to eat it.

To maximize the energy you derive from your food, be strategic about when you eat. I recommend eating at least three times a day. For optimal energy, try to eat a meal or snack roughly every three to four hours.

Eat to fuel your day. Coffee alone will not provide you with the energy or nutrients for your brain and body to function optimally. If you need your mind or body in your line of work, then it's important to feed yourself well so that you have the energy to fuel your activity.

Too many people's days are top-heavy when it comes to meals. They eat little or no breakfast, a small lunch, and as a result, they are ravenous in the afternoon and evening. We should be doing the opposite.

For optimal energy and performance, we should be front-loading our nutrition. We should eat the bulk of our calories earlier in the day to fuel our activities. The bonus is that this will result in less binge eating later in the day.

You may need to experiment to see which meal/snack strategy works best for you. Perhaps it's just three meals a day, with breakfast and lunch supplying most of your nutrition. Maybe you operate best with three meals and one snack, or three meals and two snacks. It's important to remember that, like meals, your snacks should be nutritious.

Here's an example of a three-meal, two-snack eating strategy:

- 6:30 a.m. breakfast
- 9:30 a.m. snack
- 12:30 p.m. lunch (your lunch should be larger than your dinner and eaten before 3:00 p.m.)
- 3:30 p.m. snack
- 6:30 p.m. light dinner

## Protein, Carbs, and Healthy Fat for Energy

For maximum energy and to keep hunger at bay, plan meals and snacks that contain a mix of protein, carbohydrates, and healthy fats. Here are some snack and meal options that offer a good balance of these nutrients.

**Snack Ideas**

- Apple with almond butter
- Hummus and veggies
- Roasted soy nuts
- Walnuts and grapes

**Meal Ideas**

- Oatmeal with peanut butter and one half banana
- Baked salmon with spinach and brown rice
- Beans with brown rice, broccoli, and extra virgin olive oil and Italian herbs

## Workplace Energy Strategies

Is work your home away from home? When it comes to food, work should be reminiscent of home. Try to eat as nutritiously at work as you do at home. Too much takeout, vending machine visits, and "meeting food" can take a toll on your health.

The following are some workplace strategies that can help maximize your energy, make you more productive, and keep you feeling great (and fitting into your clothes).

1. **Take movement breaks.** For more energy, incorporate movement breaks into your day. Ideally, try to spend some of these breaks outside. Moving after you eat can help regulate

your blood glucose levels. A movement break can spark creativity. Take advantage of any opportunity to move during work—an extra trip to pick up a printout, a walk to fill your water bottle, etc. Make movement a part of your regular lunchtime routine.

2. **Make your own meals and snacks.** Avoid or limit dining out and eating "meeting" food. Food prepared away from home tends to have more unsavory and/or high-calorie ingredients added. Even some of the "healthier supermarkets" use processed ingredients that include added salt or oils that aren't of the highest quality.

3. **Stay hydrated.** If you don't drink enough water, it can lead to headaches, impatience, apathy, sleepiness, and poor physical performance.[50]

4. **Ditch the candy dish.** The candy dish at work is a complete waste of time and should be eliminated from all workplaces. No one benefits from candy. It takes away from your health. It also is a trigger food for many people, meaning it can be tough to stop at one piece.

5. **Utilize Sundays and Wednesdays for meal prep.** A meal prep habit is one of the best things you can acquire this year! Consider using Sundays and Wednesdays as meal prep days. The food you make for your evening meal on Sunday can be used for Monday, Tuesday, and Wednesday's lunch meals. The food you make on Wednesday evening can be used for the Thursday and Friday meals, and Saturday, as well.

6. **Eat your fruits and vegetables.** Research has found that fruit and vegetable intake has a positive effect on well-being, curiosity, and creativity—all things we need to flourish and get the most out of a workday![51]

# Feed Your Brain

Do you nourish your brain? There are specific foods you can eat to support your mental functioning (and others that will make your brain foggy and function less optimally).

Some studies even suggest that the way you eat may influence your chances of developing dementia and Alzheimer's. The good news is that if you follow the seven recommendations below, you will be making choices that will support your brain for the long term. These strategies will help boost mental function, preserve memory, and may even help prevent Alzheimer's, dementia, and depression. What a great investment!

## Seven Simple Strategies

1. **Consider following the Mediterranean diet, and if you drink alcohol, keep it moderate.** Research has found that following the Mediterranean diet may help preserve your memory and support healthy brain function.[52] A Mediterranean diet is a way of eating that focuses on vegetables, fruits, beans, nuts, seeds, and extra virgin olive oil, while decreasing sugar, red meat, and processed foods.

   You may have seen alcohol being promoted as part of the Mediterranean diet. While there is research indicating that moderate alcohol consumption may improve quality of life as you age and may have some health benefits, there is a fine line between moderation and too much alcohol. Too much alcohol can increase your risk for cancer, stroke, heart failure, and more.

Additionally, alcohol can affect sleep. It not only can make it difficult to stay asleep, but alcohol can also lessen your REM (Rapid Eye Movement) sleep, the portion of sleep that helps you cement memories into your brain! If you do drink, sleep expert Dr. Breus recommends cutting yourself off within three hours of bedtime.[53]

2. **Eat more fish and vegetarian sources of omega-3 fatty acids.** Fish is one of those foods that offers excellent health benefits for your brain. Recent research has found that the more fish you consume, the less likely you are to develop dementia. For optimal brain function, try to eat at least eight ounces of fish per week. To make it as healthy as possible, keep fish preparation simple: maybe marinate with healthy ingredients or add a healthy dressing or light sauce to it after cooking.

The omega-3 fatty acids found in fish are important for the structure of your brain cells. They are essential fats — fats your body needs but cannot make on its own. Research has found that people with lower intakes of DHA and EPA (the omega-3 fats found in fish) have higher rates of depressive disorders.[54] If you don't eat fish, then you want to be eating the vegetarian sources of omega-3s:

**Vegetarian Sources of Omega-3 Fat**

- Ground Flaxseeds and flaxseed oil
- Walnuts and walnut oil
- Soy foods
- Hemp seeds
- Chia seeds
- Pumpkin seeds
- Organic canola oil

One important thing to note is that the omega-3 fat in fish is better absorbed than omega-3 fats from plant sources. The plant omega-3 fats need to have certain other nutrients available (such as zinc, magnesium, calcium, biotin, vitamin C, vitamin D3, and vitamin B6) in order to be converted into healthy fatty acids. So, if you are getting your omega-3s primarily from plants, it's very important to have a good baseline diet to be able to make this conversion. Too much alcohol and too many omega-6 fats (thought to be pro-inflammatory and predominant in corn oil and vegetable oil, for example) in your diet can negatively affect this conversion.

Omega-3 fats have even been found to help the brain recover after brain injury. The literature on the benefits of omega-3 fatty acids is vast and wide, but only portions of it make it to mainstream media. I started reading the literature on omega-3 fats years ago when I began writing articles for a few mental health magazines. The literature was so convincing that I added more fish and plant sources of omega-3 back into my diet. There were two things I quickly noticed in my own health: 1) The dry patches I had on my arms went away, and 2) My eyesight at night improved so much that I didn't need to wear glasses anymore while driving!

To preserve your memory (and overall good health), eat foods with omega-3 fats while limiting added sugar intake. Studies on rats have revealed that a deficiency of omega-3 fats can lead to detrimental effects on mental cognition and eating a sugar-laden diet can worsen these effects.[55]

3.  **Eat antioxidant-rich food daily.** A low intake of antioxidants in the diet is associated with cognitive impairment and Alzheimer's disease.[56] Vitamin C, beta carotene, and vitamin E are well-known antioxidants, however many plant pigments also have antioxidant effects. Vitamin C and beta carotene-rich foods may enhance your mental functioning.[57]

    You probably know that vitamin C is plentiful in citrus fruits, but it's also found in melons, such as cantaloupe and watermelon, as well as in kiwi, mango, papaya, pineapple, and most berries (like strawberries, raspberries, blueberries, and cranberries).

    Many people don't realize that vitamin C is also in sweet and white potatoes as well as other vegetables. To get a vitamin C boost, eat the following vegetables: cruciferous vegetables (like broccoli, Brussels sprouts, cabbage, and cauliflower), bell/chili peppers, and leafy greens (such as spinach, collard, and turnip greens). Tomatoes, winter squash, and okra are also excellent choices.

    Blueberries, strawberries, and spinach have been associated with improved short-term memory. What's more, blueberries may help with balance and coordination — two functions of our body that become particularly important as we age.

    Vitamin E may slow the rate of cognitive decline and reduce the risk of Alzheimer's disease.[58] Some healthful sources of vitamin E include sunflower seeds, hazelnuts, almonds, peanuts, and cooked spinach.

    The best way to ingest antioxidants is through whole foods and not pills or extracts, which may have side effects and contraindications.[59] The combination of natural bioactive components in plant foods appear to have synergistic beneficial health effects compared to when these compounds are isolated.[60]

Eat at least three servings (or more than 200 g) of vegetables per day. Antioxidants from vegetables have been associated with a lower risk of dementia and slower cognitive decline with age.[61] In particular, cruciferous vegetables, legumes, and green leafy vegetables may be helpful. Especially noteworthy vegetables are cabbage, zucchini, squash, broccoli, and leaf lettuce.[62] Garlic and the compound resveratrol, a plant chemical, may also help prevent Alzheimer's disease and cognitive decline.[63] Resveratrol is found in peanuts, pistachios, grapes, red wine, blueberries, bilberries, cranberries, and cocoa.

4.  **Eat unsaturated fats.** A higher ratio of mono and polyunsaturated fats compared with saturated fats is associated with a lower risk for mild cognitive impairment, a stage between healthy aging and dementia.[64] As a reminder, animal foods provide saturated fats, so limiting your intake of animal foods can be helpful.

5.  **Ensure adequate intake of B vitamins and vitamin D, protein, and choline.** Whole grains contain B vitamins and are particularly noteworthy for cognitive benefits. Have you switched to whole grain versions of bread, rice, cereal, and pasta? This helps provide nutrients to your body in their natural state compared with their refined counterparts, where most of the beneficial nutrients are milled away.

    Researchers have found that people who consume higher levels of folate, vitamin B6, and vitamin B12 have a lower incidence of late-life depression.[65] Vitamin D deficiency is also associated with late-life depression.[66] Dietary protein provides the amino acid tryptophan, which is needed to make serotonin, a feel-good chemical in the body that can help prevent late-life depression.[67] Dietary choline helps with the synthesis of acetylcholine in the body, which is a neurotransmitter important for memory. In Alzheimer's disease, there is a deficit of choline.[68]

Some sources of the above nutrients include:

- **Folate:** Asparagus, avocado, beans, peas, green leafy vegetables (e.g., spinach)
- **Vitamin B6:** Chickpeas, fruits (other than citrus), potatoes, salmon, tuna
- **Vitamin B12:** Dairy products, eggs, meat (limit red meat), poultry, seafood (e.g., clams, trout, salmon, haddock, tuna)
- **Choline:** egg yolk, lean top round and ground beef (limit red meat), soybeans, chicken breast, Atlantic cod, shitake mushrooms, red potatoes
- **Vitamin D:** mushrooms, wild salmon

6. **Keep caffeine intake moderate.** Research points to a protective role for coffee, tea, and other sources of caffeine. These may decrease the risk of cognitive impairment, dementia, and Alzheimer's disease.[69] More research is needed to determine optimal doses. In the meantime, moderation is key. Also, if you are having trouble sleeping, then decreasing caffeine intake may be warranted. The U.S. Dietary Guidelines lists moderate caffeine consumption as a limit of 400 mg per day (which is three to five 8-ounce cups of coffee), noting that most of the research on caffeine has been done on coffee.[70]

**The chart below compares caffeine amounts
for many popular drinks.**

| Caffeine Per Ounce in Common Caffeinated Beverages ||
|---|---|
| **Caffeinated beverage** | **Caffeine Per Ounce** |
| Drip/Brewed coffee | 12 mg/fl oz |
| Instant coffee | 8 mg/fl oz |
| Espresso | 64 mg/fl oz |
| Brewed black tea | 6 mg/fl oz |
| Brewed green tea | 2–5 mg/fl oz |
| Caffeinated soda | 1–4 mg/fl oz |
| Energy drinks | 3–35 mg/fl oz |

*Source: U.S. Dietary Guidelines[71]*

7. **Dump the diet soda.** Diet soda is one of those garbage foods that doesn't have a place in anyone's diet. Research shows there may be an association between diet soda consumption and dementia, as well as an increased risk for strokes and heart attacks.[72]

## The Importance of Sleep

Healthy habits extend beyond eating well and exercising. An important component of productivity that is often overlooked is adequate sleep. Even the best diet and exercise plans can be sabotaged by lack of sleep.

The following details habits and nutritional tips that can help improve sleep, which maximizes productivity.

## Sleep and Your Hormones

Inadequate sleep has been shown to interfere with hormone regulation, increasing your appetite, and putting you at risk for obesity and diabetes. Lack of sleep also disrupts hormone levels. You can feel hungrier because lack of sleep can drive up the hunger hormone ghrelin, and at the same time, you may feel less full because levels of the fullness hormone, leptin, are lowered.

Additionally, lack of sleep raises cortisol levels (the hormone associated with stress and belly fat) and increases insulin resistance. It also diminishes growth hormone secretion. Who wants that to happen? You lose out on the benefits of growth hormone, like protein production and fat utilization.

## Stages of Sleep

There are four stages of sleep, which are followed by the deeper Rapid Eye Movement (REM) sleep. Your body goes through several cycles of sleep stages and then REM sleep each night. Stages one and two are lighter sleep, followed by stages three and four, which are deeper sleep. A good night's rest makes you feel better physically and mentally.

According to the National Sleep Foundation, deep sleep "is when the body repairs muscles and tissues, stimulates growth and development, boosts immune function, and builds up energy for the next day."[73] REM sleep is important for memory. If you don't get enough sleep, you are jeopardizing your physical and mental health. Experts recommend seven to nine hours of sleep. Sleep hygiene (or good sleep habits) will help you get the zzzz's you need.

To get *more* and *better-quality* sleep, follow my helpful sleep tips.

## The Silverman Sleep Tight Tips

1. Have a sleep schedule. Aim for the same bedtime each night, even on weekends.

2. Eliminate caffeine, especially after 2 p.m. (some may need to eliminate it earlier or completely for best results).

3. Limit alcohol, especially three hours before bed.

4. If exercise keeps you up, exercise during the earlier part of the day.

5. Get some sun (but not too much) in the early part of the day.

6. Wind down one hour before bed. Dim the lights and turn off electronics.

7. Stay hydrated.

8. Eat a balanced and varied diet with plenty of fruits, vegetables, beans, whole grains, nuts, and seeds.

9. Eat foods rich in the following nutrients:

   - **Calcium:** Almonds, poppy seeds, yogurt, cheese, milk, fortified nondairy milks, tofu made with calcium sulfate, canned fish with edible bones (sardines, salmon, anchovies), turnip/mustard greens, broccoli, kale, okra, oranges, and calcium-fortified foods (such as orange juice and cereal)

   - **Magnesium:** Avocados, bananas, beans, peas, dairy products, green leafy vegetables (e.g., spinach), nuts, pumpkin seeds, potatoes, raisins, wheat bran, and whole grains

   - **Copper:** Chocolate (choose dark chocolate and chocolate not processed with alkali), cocoa (unsweetened cocoa powder), crustaceans and shellfish, lentils, nuts, seeds, organ meats (e.g., liver, but note that red meat should be limited), and whole grains

- **Iron:** Beans, peas, dark green vegetables, meats (red meat should be limited), poultry, prunes/prune juice, raisins, seafood, whole grain cereals, and bread

10. **Don't take sleep supplements without the guidance of a doctor.** For a natural source of the sleep hormone melatonin, eat tart cherries.

11. **Eat a carb-rich snack an hour before bed.** This is based on research from Dr. Judith Wurtman, author of *The Serotonin Solution*, which found that 25 to 35 grams of a primarily carbohydrate-based snack can increase the production of serotonin, the feel-good chemical that can contribute to good sleep.[74] Below are some examples of snacks that may help with sleep.

Please note that this snack may not be a good idea for those with diabetes, as eating carbohydrates alone, without protein and healthy fat, may spike the blood sugar.

- ¾ cup Kashi Heart to Heart Honey Toasted Oat Cereal

- 1 cup cooked old-fashioned oatmeal

- One Matthew's Whole Wheat English muffin with 1 tablespoon apple butter

- Two cups of air-popped popcorn

- Frozen whole-wheat waffle, toasted, with maple syrup

- ½ cup of whole wheat pasta topped with marinara sauce

- Four-ounce baked potato topped with salsa

Keep in mind that just as carb-rich snacks can make you sleepier, protein can have the opposite effect and make you feel more alert. It's a great idea to have a good source of protein at breakfast and lunch so that you can be alert for the day's activities. However, if you have trouble sleeping, you may want to limit your protein intake in the evening.

## NuTricia's Takeaways

Investing in getting quality sleep, timing your meals to fuel your activities, and eating foods that are linked with superior brain health will provide the wonderful healthy dividends of feeling better, thinking more clearly, and getting more done.

Here are some key takeaways:

- Aim for seven to nine hours of sleep per night.
- Limit alcohol for better sleep and mental functioning.
- Eat a rainbow of produce to boost your mental functioning.
- Eat fish and/or vegetarian sources of omega-3 fatty acids, such as walnuts, pumpkin seeds, chia seeds, and hemp seeds.
- Limit sweeteners and avoid artificial sweeteners for optimal health.
- Eat meals and snacks that contain protein, carbohydrates, and healthy fats for sustained energy during the day.

# CHAPTER 8

# Invest in Stress Management

Stressful times impact your entire life — physically, mentally, and socially. Learning to effectively manage stress is a key aspect of wellness. The vicious cycle of being stressed, eating poorly, and then sleeping poorly can be self-perpetuating. When under stress, healthy habits can help get you through the challenge. It's a matter of retraining your brain to think, "My body needs healthful food and rest when I'm stressed." At these moments, it's essential to have a few quick stress-busting options to help manage the challenge.

So many people get derailed on their wellness journey during stressful times because they have yet to find healthy strategies that work for them. My self-coaching strategies provide some healthy options. Like everything else, the most effective solution varies by individual. My list incorporates ways to manage stress and gives tips on how to motivate yourself to practice healthy habits. The goal of these strategies is to help you find healthier ways to cope with stress, so you can enjoy the dividends of feeling better, having more balance, and achieving more of your wellness goals. Review the list, try some out, and decide which ones work for you.

# NuTricia's Self-Coaching Strategies

## 1. Break the Ice on Your ...

This is one of my favorite techniques and can be used in every aspect of your life. Break the ice works really well when you're just getting started with something new, or if you're having a tough time getting started on a particular day.

Let's look at it as an exercise motivator. Imagine you have a treadmill or stationary bike at home that you have been planning to use but can't seem to get started. I invite you to break the ice on it. Breaking the ice means committing to only five or 10 minutes on that machine. Sometimes the thought of having to be on there for longer stops you from beginning. By breaking the ice, you realize that it's okay to do just a little bit. Oftentimes, it feels so good that you may continue moving longer! Go ahead, break the ice on some form of fitness that you've been planning to do!

I love the idea that just five to 10 minutes can be enough to shift your mind into gear. Some days that will be enough for the day, but on many days, it will be enough to push you forward.

## 2. Make Time for Your Energizers.

What depletes your energy? Typical answers vary, but often include finances, jobs, lack of time, health issues, relationships, etc. We all have problems; otherwise, we wouldn't be alive. Now, I want you to think about what things, specifically, make you feel happier, healthier, and more alive? These are your energizers.

Every year around the holidays, I give *Holiday Eating and Stress Reduction* seminars. I ask participants to make a list of things that make them happy (i.e., their energizers!) that don't involve food. A lot of people are so stressed that, at first, they find it hard to start the list. Take a moment and think about what these things are for you. I promise ... you have them.

A few years back, while giving a presentation at a police department, I asked the attendees what made them happy. There was an officer in the back of the room who had a stern look and stood against the wall for the entire presentation. How surprising and really nice to hear that he enjoyed writing poetry!

Other energizers people have shared with me:

- Gardening
- Walking
- Planning and taking day trips or vacations
- Spending time with family and friends
- Taking pictures of nature
- Live performances and events such as music, comedy, theater, and sports
- Reading (My favorite genre to read is memoir. If I don't have one next to my bed, I feel like I am missing something. What are your favorite types of books?)
- Massages, facials
- Dancing

**Write your top five energizers here. Aim to incorporate at least one of these into your calendar over the next two weeks.**

1.
2.
3.
4.
5.

## 3. Be Accountable.

Accountability ensures change happens. It's the difference between wanting to make a change and committing to it. You set specific goals, tell someone who will support you what they are, and enlist their help. Your accountability partner can be a coach, dietitian, trainer, friend, partner, or yourself. Just make it someone who's ready to look out for you!

Accountability can lead to weight loss success. If you choose to be accountable to yourself and you are looking for weight loss, weigh in at least once per week, and not multiple times per day. I have numerous success stories with varying intervals of weighing in. Find what works for you and don't obsess about it because a variety of things can alter the scale, including monthly cycles, what you recently ate, and when you went to the bathroom last. I find it best to weigh myself first thing in the morning. One strategy that worked for me while getting rid of the weight I gained during pregnancies was to weigh in every Friday and then again on Monday. Weighing in on Friday helped me to stay motivated over the weekend and weighing in on Monday helped me to get back on track if I fell off. Some clients I have worked with have found it helpful to weigh in on a daily basis.

## 4. Set an Imaginary Alarm.

Along with weighing in periodically, you might want to set an imaginary alarm system for your weight. I have a weight that if I hit, the alarms go off. It gets me right back on track doing all of the strategies I share in this book. These strategies have helped me and the people I have coached, as well as many others, get and stay healthy and fit.

What is your alarm system number? 120, 130, 150, 180, 200 pounds, or another number? The alarm is unique to each individual. Set it. It works like a charm!

## 5. Practice Mindfulness, Meditation, and Yoga.

Managing stress and practicing wellness does not always involve big movements or actions. Sometimes, you need to find quieter moments where you can pause and escape from the constant barrage of technology (calls, emails, social media, and texts). By unplugging and adding quiet contemplation into your day, you'll discover greater focus and a more peaceful you.

Here are my three favorite ways to quiet my mind.

**Mindfulness** can help you to manage stress, eat better, lose weight, and achieve your goals. Mindfulness is the "tuning in" or "paying attention" to what is going on in the moment. I shared about mindful eating earlier in the book. This is when you remove distractions, such as reading, cell phones, or the TV, and focus on what you are eating.

People who use food to cope, often use it to "tune out." Tuning in makes you more aware of what you are doing, and what is serving you (and what isn't). Breathing techniques, meditation, and yoga all use mindfulness.

**Meditation** comes in many forms. Meditation can help you to get in better control of your thoughts and actions. In their book, *Real Meditation in Minutes a Day*, Joseph Arpaia and Lobsang Rapgay describe meditation as "exercise for the mind."[75] Meditation practices vary but may include breathing exercises, guided meditations that take you on peaceful mind journeys, progressive relaxation meditations that relax you from head to toe by tensing then releasing muscles, and more.

If you are a beginner, consider starting with three to five minutes of a form of meditation that appeals to you. Insight Timer is a great free meditation app. There is an upgrade fee if you want added functions, such as fast-forward and rewind. Calm and Headspace are other popular meditation apps, and fees vary. Gaiam offers a free downloadable meditation. Deepak Chopra and Oprah often offer free 21-day meditation options. You can sign up here to be alerted of future offerings or to purchase past programs: ChopraCenterMeditation. com/. There are also helpful free meditation downloads here: https://www.uclahealth.org/Marc/Mindful-Meditations.

**Yoga** can be viewed as moving meditation. One of the best ways to self-coach yourself for wellness and weight loss is to develop a yoga practice. Yoga can help you to lose weight practically effortlessly. People who have lost weight through yoga often report that their waist is noticeably thinner. This may be because the size of your waist often reflects the size of your stress (I heard this from Dr. Oz a while back! What a helpful visual!). And yoga is a known stress reliever.

Yoga can also have a big impact on your eating habits by making you feel less hungry. Combining movement and mindfulness makes it easier to practice mindful eating. It also encourages healthier eating habits. Practicing yoga is a great way to cope with anxiety, boredom, or depression. Twisting poses and headstands seem to be particularly helpful.[76] And don't worry if the thought of a headstand gives you a headache—there are other poses that can give you similar benefits.

## 6. Use Spirituality to Help Guide Your Wellness.

**Pray, and pray some more!** Pray to whomever you want — to god, your ancestors, or your "higher power," as they say in group recovery programs. Pray for health, help, love, and success.

Over the past few years, I have started to learn more about the wellness habits of longevity cultures, such as the Okinawans. For the Okinawans, prayer is important, and they often pray to their ancestors. After reading about them, I pray to my own ancestors, and have really felt more peace and a guiding presence since doing so.

## 7. Use Music to Lift You Up and Motivate You to Move.

There's nothing like listening to music from your teen years to help lift your spirits and get you motivated to move! Classical music has been studied for its numerous wellness benefits. It may help to reduce your stress and anxiety and boost your mood and creativity!

In cultures of longevity, singing, music, and dance seem to play a role in lengthening the lifespan.

## 8. Take a Library Stroll.

This is one of my favorite "techniques," and one I love to share because it brings an element of the unexpected into your life. A library stroll means taking a walk through the aisles of the library and discovering books, hobbies, concepts, and resources you never knew existed. You can do this in one section of the library or wander the entire library. There's one particularly lonely part of the library waiting for you to visit … that's the cookbook section. My strolls there have gifted me wonderful recipes and have sparked creativity for my own recipes. Go take a stroll and see what you discover!

## 9. Employ Self-Coping Strategies.

How we cope can strengthen us or further zap our energy. If we find ourselves coping with stress by using food, alcohol, drugs, or gambling, then we need to take a step back and identify which self-coping strategies we have that are not helping us, and consider why we're using them. Once we know what we turn to when we're struggling, we can start changing habits and establishing new responses that serve us better. Many of the other ideas on this list can serve as coping strategies, like yoga, fitness, and energizers. Below are a few others that I have found particularly helpful.

**Tapping or emotional freedom technique (EFT)** is a method of coping that uses affirmations along with tapping on the meridians of the body used in acupuncture. I have used it to ease feelings of tension and anxiety. I learned how to do it by watching Julie Schiffman's videos. Julie, Expert EFT Practitioner and Certified Emotion Code Practitioner/ Body Code Practitioner, has been kind enough to let me show one of her videos in my *Self-Coaching Strategies for Wellness and Weight Loss* presentations. You can find her videos at JulieSchiffman.com. Julie has shared her passion for EFT with me and explains, "EFT/ tapping is an amazing technique. I am so grateful for it every day as I see so many lives being transformed (even my own)."

**Gratitude** is being appreciative for what you have rather than focusing on what you don't have. Thinking or journaling about what you are grateful for upon awakening can help give you a more positive mind-set to start off the day. Some people prefer to reflect on what they're grateful for in the evening before bed, perhaps writing a few things in a gratitude journal to remind them of the positive parts of their day.

When I practice gratitude, I think about how I am grateful for hugs from my children, support from my husband, the way the light hits the ground in the pre-sunset hours, sunsets, and for the people who have believed in me and have been kind to me.

**Forgiveness** can help you put the past in the past so that you can move on to a more positive mind-set. I particularly like Everett Worthington's Reach for Forgiveness technique:[77]

Recall the Hurt

Empathize (put yourself in the other person's shoes; try to see it their way)

Altruistic gift (give an unselfish gift of forgiveness)

Commit to forgiveness (write yourself a note committing to forgiveness)

Hold onto forgiveness (keep the note to remind yourself you forgave)

**Self-compassion** is another framework that I've found to be extremely helpful. It was developed by Dr. Kristin Neff and relies on three guiding principles:[78]

1. **Self-Kindness:** Treat yourself with kindness, as you would a friend.
2. **Common Humanity:** Know that you aren't alone. Others are going through similar situations.
3. **Mindfulness:** Be more positive than negative about situations.

Self-compassion also includes soothing touch. An example of soothing touch is to take your hand and give your opposite arm a gentle squeeze. Another form of soothing touch is to cross your hands over your heart and feel the gentle warmth that starts to radiate. Your body can't distinguish who is giving the touches, so you get similar benefits to when a mom holds a baby.

## 10. Have a Plan.

A really helpful way to stay focused on wellness involves making a plan. At the beginning of the week, decide what you're going to cook, when you're going to shop, and which days you'll work out.

For instance, some of my clients find it helpful to spend Sunday planning meals for the week and shopping for ingredients. Then, they may cook on Monday, eat leftovers on Tuesday and Wednesday (which makes these good days to take fitness classes), and then cook again on Thursday. When cooking on Monday and Thursday, they prepare larger batches of food, so there's a reserve of healthy foods to select from for meals before you have to cook again. Pick which days work best for you to batch-cook!

## 11. Move Along the Stage of Change.

Realize that when it comes to changing behaviors, there is a helpful framework that can help you discover where you may be stuck and give some direction to where you want to go.

The framework is Prochaska and DiClemente's Stages of Change Model summarized in the bullets below.[79] As we look through the stages, let's use the example of a person in their 40s who has gained 100 pounds since high school.

- Pre-contemplation (Not Ready for Change) The person isn't looking to lose weight. It's not even on their radar.
- Contemplation (Thinking About Change) The person is thinking about losing weight.
- Preparation (Preparing for Action) The person has researched the WW (formerly Weight Watcher's) program, a weight loss challenge program at work, and the Paleo Diet.
- Action (Taking Action) The person signs up for the challenge at work and starts logging her food into MyFitnessPal.
- Maintenance (Maintaining a Good Behavior) The person lost 85 pounds and is now maintaining that weight by logging her

food at least three times per week, eating more vegetables, and watching portion size.

If you are stuck in a stage of change, then try listing the pros and cons of entering the next stage. The pros usually outweigh the cons, which can be motivating and helpful in moving to the next stage.

## 12. Practice Self-Efficacy.

Self-efficacy is the belief that you are able to start and maintain a desired behavior. There are personal, environmental, and behavioral factors that can support self-efficacy:

**Personal:** Do more things that recharge you (i.e., your energizers, such as reading, sight-seeing, massage, hot bath).

**Environmental:** Surround yourself with people who are successful at what you are trying to achieve, and those who give you motivation (exercise class instructor, coach, trainer, mentor, and supportive friend).

**Behavioral:** Set small goals that are achievable, such as focusing on making one meal healthier this week, or getting 10 minutes of exercise today.

## 13. Have a Vision.

After determining which of the self-coaching strategies best suits you, it's time to look at the big picture. Making good choices on a daily basis is important, but you also need a longer term vision of where you want to be and what you want to accomplish. The easiest way to attain goals is by setting them. Vision boards help with this by clarifying what you want to achieve and setting the direction.

## Using a Vision Board

Creating a vision board is a way to help "clarify, concentrate, and maintain focus on a specific life goal," according to MakeAVisionboard.com.[80] A vision board is a place where you gather and display images that portray what you want to do, be, have, or aspire to in your life. Here is a vision board I developed a few years back. It's amazing how many things have come to fruition.

## Tricia's Vision Board

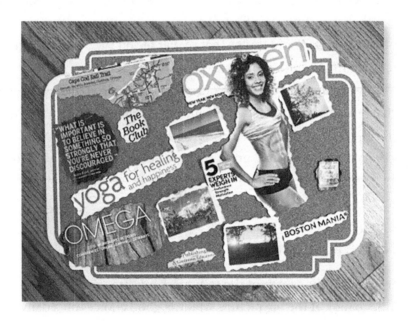

Now is a good time for you to create your vision board. Remember, it's meant to inspire you to attain a dream. It's meant to be a visual tool to help you stay focused on your goals. A great resource to help you get started can be found at MakeAVisionBoard.com.

## Write Your Vision Down

In addition to (or instead of) creating a vision board, writing your vision down can be very effective too. It's helpful to create a written vision of where you want to be in a specific period of time (for example, three months). You write it as if you are already living that way in the future.

Here is a sample vision.

Three months from now, I weigh eight pounds less. I sleep at least seven hours per night. I turn off my computer and phone by 10:30 p.m. each night. I feel energized. I weigh myself every Friday and Monday. I spend at least 30 minutes per week decluttering. I walk five days a week for at least 30 minutes each. I do two days of strength training per week. I have tried at least one gentle yoga class by this time. I get a facial every 90 days. I visit or plan a visit to my adult children every four months. I go on date nights with my partner every two weeks. I try two new recipes each month.

This is a great start and focuses on measurable actions. Now, it's time to create your vision. Consider the following questions:

- What do you want to be doing in three months from now?
- How do you want to be feeling?
- How much do you want to be exercising?
- What do you want your fitness to look like?
- What other elements from the book do you want to be doing?

Write your vision in the present tense. Once your vision is complete, it's time to set goals to help you get to that vision. Write your vision here:

# 14. Set Your Goals.

Written goals are more apt to happen. Set weekly or monthly process goals to help you attain your vision.

When setting goals, the following SMART acronym is helpful:

**S-pecific:** Be specific about your goals. For instance, I want to lose weight is too vague. I want to lose 10 pounds is specific.

**M-easurable:** Put a measurable component within your goals, such as I will log my food five out of seven days.

**A-ttainable:** Make sure your goals are attainable. If you said you wanted to lose 15 pounds in one week, that's not attainable, but one or two pounds is.

**R-easonable:** Reasonable goals are more likely to be accomplished. Saying you will work out every day for a month is not reasonable, however saying five or more days per week is.

**T-ime bound:** Putting a time or date on your goal makes it more likely to happen.

## What are your 30-year goals?

For years, I've been setting yearly, weekly, and daily goals. Then I heard international motivational speaker and fitness expert, Sergeant Ken Weichert, recommend setting 30-year goals. This gave me a whole new perspective. Many of us have 30-year mortgages, so why not have a 30-year vision and 30-year goals?

What goals would you like to set to help you get to your vision? Here is an example that corresponds to the sample vision above:

This week I will:

1. Log my food into a food logging app at least five out of the next seven days.
2. I will walk 15 minutes per day at least four days of my work week and one day on the weekend.
3. I will try a new salad recipe on Saturday.
4. On Saturday, I will research local yoga studios to find a gentle yoga class to take over the next month.
5. I will book a facial for the end of the month

List 1-5 goals here that you will work on this week.

1.

2.

3.

4.

5.

Having a daily to-do list can help you reach your goals and get more things done.

## NuTricia's Takeaways

These strategies include ways to coach you through your stress and how to motivate yourself to practice healthy habits. Taking care of yourself allows you to enjoy the dividends of feeling better, having more balance, and achieving more of your wellness goals.

Here are key takeaways:

- Make time for your energizers.
- Set a weight alarm to sound off to help keep your weight down.
- Practice mindfulness, meditation, and yoga.
- Bring more spirituality into your life.
- Use music to motivate you.
- Practice forgiveness and gratitude.
- Have a plan. Create a vision board, a written vision, and written goals.

# CHAPTER 9

# Taking the Next Step to Wellness

As you can see, longevity and wellness can be impacted by a variety of factors: nutrition, fitness and weight management, and healthy lifestyle habits. If you incorporate even small changes, you will likely reap noticeable dividends.

There is one final piece of the puzzle that can help ensure your success, and that is finding purpose.

## Finding Your Purpose

Finding a sense of purpose is an often overlooked element of overall health. One reason for this connection with health may be that when we have a purpose, we're more likely to take care of ourselves—to implement all the principles we've discussed in this book. And it's possible that making all those little, positive choices creates new purpose which leads us to better physical and mental health, and leads to longevity.

But interestingly, research indicates there is also evidence that having a sense of purpose alone may have a powerful effect on health, well-being, and longevity. And the best news? It doesn't seem to matter if you don't find your purpose until late in life.

While the exact reasons for this are unclear, researchers suspect that individuals who have a sense of purpose have a more positive outlook. Taking part in meaningful activities makes us happy and reduces stress. This is linked to lower levels of cortisol, which is beneficial for brain function and the immune system.[81]

## What Do You Want to Do When You "Retire"?

Many people are working and dreaming of their retirement. However, people in some cultures of longevity (such as Okinawa) do not even have a word for retirement. Artie Carey is in his 70s and still working alongside his son for the plumbing company they own in Needham, Massachusetts. Artie started to notice the demise of some of his friends after they retired—some who were still in their 60s. They had lost their purpose.

Whether or not you retire, it's important for your longevity to have a purpose. When asked if he was going to retire, it seemed like Artie had no intention of doing so when he laughed and replied, "Maybe in my 80s." Read the story about Nan McEvoy below. She started a whole new career in her 70s. I stumbled upon her inspiring story when I toured the McEvoy Ranch orchards and olive oil mill in a quest to learn more about extra virgin olive oil.

### Add Years to Your Life with a Purpose

Nan McEvoy developed a whole new business when she retired. Nan's grandfather was a founder of the *San Francisco Chronicle*. She was destined to be a socialite, but instead wrote for the Chronicle and then moved to the East Coast where she worked for the *New*

*York Herald Tribune* and the *Washington Post.* She returned to the *Chronicle* and headed the board from 1981 to 1995. She came across a beautiful property in Petaluma, California, and founded McEvoy Ranch there in 1991, before she retired from the Chronicle.

She worked with an olive oil expert from Italy to develop the land into an olive tree oasis. One of the beautiful features of the property is a Chinese pagoda that Nan had built, which can be rented out for functions. Another visual feast for the eyes – besides the thousands of olive oil trees – are the gardens built into the hillside.

Nan grew this business into a thriving organic olive oil company that also sells wine and products made from olive oil. She is also responsible for bringing in the olive trees from Italy that helped many other California producers get their start in the industry. Nan passed away at 95-years-old. What an amazing contribution she made to organic agriculture in her golden years! To learn more about Nan's legacy and where to buy the McEvoy Ranch olive oil, check out their website at McEvoyRanch.com.

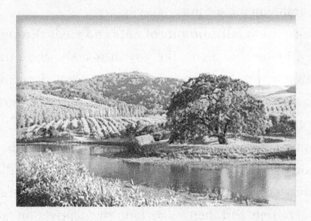

*Photo credit: Courtesy of McEvoy Ranch*

## NuTricia's Tips for a Long, Healthy Life

Getting started on a healthy path is sometimes the hardest part, and you may be wondering how to begin. Below is a summary of some of the steps you can take to ensure you live the longest, healthiest life possible.

Which of these strategies will you adopt as your investments to reap the dividends of a longer, stronger life? The more of these you incorporate, the better you will feel and be!

1. **Eat lots of vegetables! Whenever possible, eat vegetables and fruits that are in season and locally grown. Garden if you can and/or try to purchase foods from local farm stands and farmers' markets. When steaming or boiling vegetables, consume the leftover water.** The water that remains from steaming zucchini makes a tasty vegetable tea. When you cook vegetables, you lose some of the nutrients in the water. That water is liquid platinum! It's chock-full of nutrients and can be a nice healthy way to end a meal, instead of grabbing for seconds.

2. **Consume small amounts of nuts and seeds throughout the day.** Remember Ken? The guy in his 90s who came to my seminar with his "young" girlfriend? He had nuts with him that were his snack for the day. However, watch portion size! Nuts are very calorie dense.

3. **Limit your red meat consumption. Eat more beans. Eat more fish.** Too many people keep jumping on fad diets to get short-term results. Then they go off the diet for cheat days or cheat meals and then go back on the deprivation fad diet — until they go back off again. It's much better to move toward having an overall philosophy of healthy eating.

For instance, the current keto diet fad severely restricts carbs and encourages people **not** to eat fruit. Fruit is nature's candy and, among other health benefits, can help prevent cancer and macular degeneration (yes, this means better eye health for you if you eat your fruit!). The Paleo diet discourages beans. Beans are a staple in longevity cultures. They help to lower cholesterol levels, and prevent constipation! Fad diets are often shortsighted and don't prepare people for long-term health. Think more about eating for both the short and the long term.

4. **Decrease processed food consumption. Try fruit when you crave sweet treats.** Eating healthy fruits is what they do in many longevity cultures, rather than choosing candy or baked treats. Next time you crave something sweet, try a cup of frozen cherries (dark, sweet cherries or combined with tart cherries) dusted with unsweetened cocoa powder. Nips a craving right in the bud.

5. **Stay active and move your body regularly.** Whether you take classes at the gym or walk outside during your lunch break, the key to staying active is finding the type of movement that you like to do. This keeps you motivated and committed to moving on a regular schedule. To discover what you like to do, it may be helpful to set periodic short-term goals that involve trying new fitness activities, such as a yoga or Pilates class.

6. **Stay connected to family and friends.** In Okinawa, they have moais, which are groups of people that get together for social and financial support. The *Okinawa Program* describes a group of guys who went to kindergarten together. They were still getting together in their 80s.[82] What if you don't

have family near you? Joining clubs is a great way to meet people and make new connections, no matter your age.

Remember Artie the plumber from earlier in the chapter? One of the ways he stays connected to his family is that he works with his son. I've gotten to know Artie and his son pretty well over the years, and they have a special relationship. Artie says it well, "He's my best friend." Continuing to work in his 70s and working with his son gives him purpose (see number 7).

7. **Have a purpose.** What is your purpose? What are your unique gifts? Are you using them now? How can you use them when and if you retire? One way is through volunteerism. An active ager I met at a senior center spends her time volunteering at a nursing home where she visits patients. It gives her purpose and joy to visit with people who may no longer get social visits from anyone else.

## Finding Purpose in a Second Career

Terry DeAngelis is a spunky trainer and fitness competition coach with a contagiously positive attitude. She has amassed an unbelievable amount of training strategies over the last 30 years. People who keep physically active seem to age slower than their sedentary counterparts, and Terry is a great example of this.

She moves around and has the energy of a 20-year-old. Like Nan and her olive trees, Terry has found her purpose. This is a second career for her. She is a retired flight attendant and began competing in bodybuilding competitions while she was still flying in the 1980s. Terry's purpose is to continue learning, so she can give her clients the best strategies and protocols to reach their goals. She loves how getting ready for fitness competitions allows women of any age to get excited about an event and likens it to getting ready for prom. She loves to help women feel inner and outer beauty, embrace themselves, and be gorgeous.

8.  **Aim to be happy and cheerful.** Terry, from the story above, is always happy and cheerful. To keep life fun, Terry maintains a balanced life that includes social time with her friends as well as time spent on herself. She works on her inner self by meditating every morning to contemplate and sort out how she is feeling. This gives her the faith that she will *know* what she needs to do moving forward for the day.

    Reading books by Norman Vincent Peale, Zig Ziglar, and Ken Blanchard helped me go from a negative to more positive outlook during my college years. Norman Vincent Peale's books actually brought my husband and me closer while dating — so much so, to my mother's initial disappointment, we gave away his *Power of Positive Thinking* books as our wedding favors. (The idea eventually grew on her, and she wrapped them up beautifully!)

    Lately, I am gobbling up motivational books by Brian Tracy. My clients have enjoyed reading his *Eat the Frog* book. Another favorite is Tracy's *Get Smart: How to Think and Act Like the Most Successful and Highest-Paid People in Every Field.*

9.  **Embrace spirituality.** Spirituality can be (but doesn't have to be) organized religion. It can be any religion or philosophy that gets you in touch with a higher or inner source of guidance and peace. Terry's spirituality has grown, and one of her prayers is to ask for help to *do* what she needs to do.

10. **Minimize exposure to chemicals in your food and in the products you use on your body and in your home.** Consider buying more natural and organic foods, and foods with the shortest ingredient lists. If the ingredients listed are not ones that are available for you to purchase (not that you would want to!) and store in your cabinet (such as BHT), then you are probably better off without them. Use more natural products, and open a window to get more air circulating in your house when you vacuum and use chemicals. Synthetic products you may be using on your body, skin, and hair may be wreaking havoc and causing reactions in your body.

We also should take time to celebrate achievement of our goals. You have one achievement to celebrate now... finishing the book! Congratulations! Enjoy your dividends.

> ## Thank you for reading *Healthy Dividends!*
>
> ### Word-of-mouth is really helpful for getting the word out about my book. Please consider submitting a brief review wherever you can.

# Appendix A

## Longevity Cultures

There are regions of longevity across the world where people thrive in their older years without the high rates of cancer, heart disease, diabetes, and dementia that affect many Americans in their later years. Dan Buettner joined forces with *National Geographic* and has written books about the people of some of these regions and their lifestyle habits.[83] He calls these areas "Blue Zones" and has started developing new Blue Zones in the United States. We already had one, Loma Linda, California, which I had the good fortune of visiting in 2017. In his book, he highlights his travels to the Blue Zones of Costa Rica, Loma Linda, Italy, Greece, and Okinawa.

What many people don't know is that *National Geographic* magazine teamed up with another researcher in the early 1970's to learn more about the people in areas known for longevity at that time. Dr. Alexander Leaf of Harvard Medical School visited Hunza (in northern Pakistan), Abkhazia (part of the former Soviet Union), and Vilcabamba (in Ecuador).[84]

At the time, people were claiming to live well beyond 120 years.[85] Not long after, age exaggeration in some cultures of longevity was revealed.[86] The reasons for this exaggeration range from family, religious, or national pride to pension fraud and documentation fraud from earlier years (resulting from an effort to avoid or get into the military).[87]

Mainstream interest in extreme longevity seemed to diminish as a result of the age exaggeration debacle until Dan Buettner breathed new air into it. Even though the reality of age exaggeration was proven to be true, it should be remembered that older adults were thriving in certain cultures, without many of the diseases and afflictions we attribute to old age. There are many lessons to be learned from those still healthy in old age.

The following are observations and tips from various longevity cultures. Abkhazia, Vilcabamba, Hunza, and Okinawa are discussed extensively by John Robbins in his book, *Healthy at 100*.[88] Costa Rica, Loma Linda, the Mediterranean, and Okinawa are discussed in *Blue Zones* and *Blue Zones Solution* by Dan Buettner.[89] Two books that are really wonderful at explaining the Okinawan diet and lifestyle that lends itself to longevity are *The Okinawa Way* and *The Okinawa Diet Plan*.

## Abkhazia

One attendee of one of my employee wellness programs was of Abkhazian descent. She described how the various generations of her family in Abkhazia lived together. In many areas of longevity, several generations of the family live together so the grandparents and great-grandparents may help with the child-rearing duties of the grandchildren and great-grandchildren.

An interesting food habit that would be worthwhile for you to consider is the Abkhazian's breakfast of salad and a cornmeal porridge.[90] Eating raw vegetables is common in areas of longevity. Not surprisingly, research has shown that a high fruit, vegetable, and bean (legume) intake decreases mortality, compared with a low consumption rate.[91] Raw vegetables are particularly important for longevity. Nuts are featured in the cuisine of longevity cultures.

## Vilcabamba, Ecuador

Jon Robbins shared that in Vilcabamba, there is a popular saying which refers to the power of walking, "You have two doctors, your left leg, and your right leg."[92] People in areas of longevity tend to do a lot of low impact physical activity such as walking, dancing, tai chi, tending the land (pruning trees, gardening, removing brush), and tending to animals.

## Hunza, Pakistan

Hunza, Pakistan, is a region known for its beautiful, organic, terraced gardens. It helped spark the organic movement in the United States. J. I. Rodale, the publisher of *Organic Gardening Magazine,* and many other healthy publications was fascinated by Hunzan farming techniques. Rodale wrote about the healthy ways of the people of Hunza in his 1949 book titled, *The Healthy Hunzas.*[93]

In June 1958, Dr. Alexander Banik, an optometrist, visited Hunza and wrote the book *Hunza Land* about his travels.[94] Dr. Banik was a fan of Art Linkletter's *People are Funny* show and wrote to the producers suggesting they should send someone to Hunza to learn and then share about the Hunzan lifestyle with Americans. His interest in Hunza stemmed from a magazine article he read touting the "extraordinary health and vigor" of the Hunzans.[95] The show ended up sending Dr. Banik to Hunza!

How can you eat more like the Hunzans? Eat more raw fruits and vegetables for sure! Apricots and mulberries are popular in Hunza and are eaten dried when they are not in season.[96] You can purchase Hunzan dried mulberries and golden raisins at Whole Foods. They are also available online with Hunzan Goji berries at https://internationalharvest.com/. Banik reported that people in Hunza primarily ate fruits, vegetables, beans, goat milk and cheese, and walnuts.[97] Walnuts contain the brain and heart health-boosting omega-3 fats! Meat and egg consumption are rare in the traditional Hunzan diet.

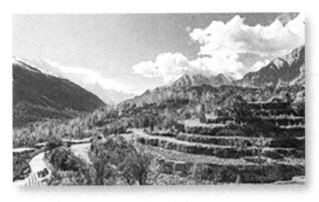

*Terraced Garden in Hunza, Pakistan. Source: Pixabay*

## Nicoya Peninsula, Costa Rica

In the Nicoya peninsula area of Costa Rica, they eat a lighter evening meal, as opposed to meals in the United States where people tend to have a top-heavy day when it comes to food consumption.[98] Practicing eating lighter as the day goes on can help support weight loss.

## Loma Linda, California

Loma Linda has a high population of Seventh Day Adventists. Healthy eating and attention to wellness are cornerstones of this religion. Followers are often plant-based eaters, and they avoid alcohol, coffee, and cigarettes.

During my visit to Loma Linda, I asked community members, hotel staff, and members of the Loma Linda Senior Center, "Why do people live such long, healthy lives in Loma Linda?" Everyone shared that the same two factors were responsible. Can you guess? Diet (no surprise) … and religion! A nutrition presentation by professor Hans Diehl at the Loma Linda University Church was very telling of the culture of Loma Linda: references to God were frequently brought into the discussion. This was something I've never witnessed at a nutrition program. It was very inspiring! How impressive that Loma Linda Senior Center has a vegetarian menu in addition to its regular menu!

## Okinawa, Japan

Okinawa is a series of islands off the southwest coast of Japan. It is part of Japan but has ties from the past to both Japan and China, which are reflected in its customs. Okinawa is known for its high population of centenarians. Okinawans enjoy a mostly plant-based diet. Hara Hachi Bu is their practice of eating until they are only 80% full, which is basically eating until you are gently satisfied, but not full.[99] You're probably wondering, "How do I do this?" It's simple. Leave some room in your belly after you eat. Don't eat to complete fullness.

Faith is a part of the healing practice in Okinawa. If you are sick, you might visit both a traditional medical doctor and a shaman (spiritual healer) as well. One of the staple Okinawan foods is the imo, a purple yam (white on the outside), available at Asian supermarkets in the United States. Go to https://www.triciasilverman.com/book for a delicious, healthy recipe where you can use either a Japanese yam or a sweet potato. The recipe was created by award-winning Chef, Steve Uliss, with some input from yours truly.

## The Mediterranean Region

The Epic Study researchers in Greece found that the Mediterranean diet is associated with lower mortality, meaning it may help you live longer! They monitored over 28,000 people and found the following particularly helpful:[100]

- low intake of meat/meat products
- high intake of vegetables, fruits and nuts, olive oil, and legumes
- moderate intake of alcohol

The Mediterranean Diet promotes eating abundant colorful fruits and vegetables, whole grains, and beans. An easy way to follow this diet is to shop for a rainbow when you are in the produce aisle. Fat is mostly in the form of nuts, seeds, and extra virgin olive oil. Physical activity is a cornerstone of the Mediterranean lifestyle. What's more, the Mediterranean Diet may improve your cognition and memory and reduce the risk for dementia.[101] Whole grains and fish may be especially advantageous.[102]

Red wine in moderation is also a well-known feature of this diet. However, if you don't consume alcohol, don't start. There are so many other habits in this book that I hope you will try instead. See more on alcohol, including guidelines for moderation in chapter 6.

# Appendix B

## NuTricia's Meal Plan

I created the 1,600-calorie meal plan below for people in order to show them how to balance their food choices throughout the day. The chart gives a big picture view of the types of decisions and choices you have when going through a typical day.

The Meal Plan takes into account and simplifies food groupings made popular by the USDA's former food pyramid and current MyPlate, as well as the Exchange System developed by the American Diabetes Association and the Academy of Nutrition and Dietetics.[103] Here is a description of the meal plan:

- In the first column, the meal plan outlines five different meal occasions, spaced throughout the day.
- In column two, I detail the number of servings from specified food groups for each meal.
- In column three, sample foods and suggested menus are listed. If you don't like the foods listed, you can swap them out for your preferred foods in that particular food group. For instance, if you don't like oatmeal, you can swap it out for another food from the starch food group, such as dry cereal.

Examples of items in each food group category can be found in the pages after the meal plan.

- In the next columns, the days of the week are listed with blank spaces beneath. Here, you can write in the foods you eat each day.

- At the bottom of the table, there is a section called Number of Choices and Serving Size. This section breaks down food groups into servings, so you can track what you are eating in each food group. As you add a food to the table, you should also fill in the bubble at the bottom of the sheet. If, at the end of the day, you are still hungry, look for empty bubbles. Let's say two fat bubbles were empty. This means you can eat two servings from the fat group. Since six almonds equal one serving, perhaps you will have 12 almonds.

Note: To the left of the bubble columns, it tells you the total number of choices for each food group for the day.

- At the end of the dinner meal, notice that it lists two Carbs, and the column to the right says 160 calories. This allows you to choose either two carb servings (a carb serving is either a fruit, a starch, or a milk group serving), or 160 calories of whatever you prefer. These calories are listed as discretionary calories in the bubble area of the meal plan. Perhaps you want to have more protein. If so, then you can add 160 calories of chicken, fish, or beans. And they don't have to be at dinner — you can tack on these extra calories wherever you want them. You also can use these 160 calories toward a small indulgence such as dark chocolate.

- Below the discretionary calories is an area where you can fill in bubbles to monitor how much water you're drinking. As close to eight glasses of water a day is best. The bubbles are a good reminder to stay hydrated. There's also an area where you can note your exercise as well.

If you want a meal plan for a different calorie level and access to more comprehensive food lists, please consider coaching with me! You can contact me through my website at **https://www.triciasilverman.com/contact**.

## Sample 1600 Calorie Meal Plan

| | Number of Servings | Menu Ideas | Day 1 | Day 2 | Day 3 | Day 4 | Day 5 | Day 6 | Day 7 |
|---|---|---|---|---|---|---|---|---|---|
| When you get up | 1 Starch<br>1 cup Milk<br>1 Fruit<br>1 Fat | ½ cup cooked oatmeal<br>1 cup skim milk<br>1 small banana (4 oz.)<br>4 walnut halves | | | | | | | |
| Mid-morning snack | 1.5 cup Milk<br>1 Fruit<br>1 Fat | 1 cup 0% Fage plain yogurt<br>2 Tbsp. or 1 minibox raisins<br>½ Tbsp. cashew butter | | | | | | | |
| Lunch-time | 2 Starch<br>1 Vegetable<br>.5 Vegetable<br>2.5 Lean Protein<br>2 Fat | ⅔ cup brown rice<br>1 cup salad greens<br>.5 cup cucumber<br>2.5 oz. tuna<br>2 tsp. extra virgin olive oil | | | | | | | |
| Mid-afternoon snack | 1 Fruit<br>1 Fat<br>1 Lean Protein | 1 small apple<br>½ Tbsp. peanut butter<br>1 oz. light cheese | | | | | | | |
| Dinner and Dessert | 2 Starch<br>.5 Vegetable<br>1 Vegetable<br>1 Fat<br>3 Lean Protein<br>2 Carb | ⅔ cup whole wheat pasta<br>.5 cup cabbage slaw<br>.5 cup steamed broccoli<br>1 tsp. organic canola oil<br>3 oz. chicken<br>160 calorie snack | | | | | | | |
| Number of Choices and Serving Size: | 3 | Fruit ½ cup | ○○○ | ○○○ | ○○○ | ○○○ | ○○○ | ○○○ | ○○○ |
| | 3 | Veg. ½ c. cooked 1 c. raw | ○○○ | ○○○ | ○○○ | ○○○ | ○○○ | ○○○ | ○○○ |
| | 5 | Starch oz. | ○○○○○ | ○○○○○ | ○○○○○ | ○○○○○ | ○○○○○ | ○○○○○ | ○○○○○ |
| | 6.5 | Meats/Beans/Cheese oz. | ○○○○○○⊖ | ○○○○○○⊖ | ○○○○○○⊖ | ○○○○○○⊖ | ○○○○○○⊖ | ○○○○○○⊖ | ○○○○○○⊖ |
| | 2.5 | Milk 8 oz. cup | ○○⊖ | ○○⊖ | ○○⊖ | ○○⊖ | ○○⊖ | ○○⊖ | ○○⊖ |
| | 6 | Fats tsp. | ○○○○○○ | ○○○○○○ | ○○○○○○ | ○○○○○○ | ○○○○○○ | ○○○○○○ | ○○○○○○ |
| | | 160 discretionary calories | | | | | | | |
| | 8 | Water 8 oz. cup | ○○○○○<br>○○○ | ○○○○○<br>○○○ | ○○○○○<br>○○○ | ○○○○○<br>○○○ | ○○○○○<br>○○○ | ○○○○○<br>○○○ | ○○○○○<br>○○○ |
| | | Exercise | | | | | | | |

# NuTricia's Food Groupings and Calories

The following groupings divide food into fruit, non-starchy vegetables, starch, protein, milk, and fat. There are also free foods. If you are trying to figure out how many servings you are eating, notice the calories per serving noted at the top of each group and use a food scale and/or measuring cups to help you estimate.

## Fruit

**One serving equals 60 calories.**

**In general, one serving is one small piece of fruit, or approximately one half cup of fresh fruit or two tablespoons of dried fruit or half cup unsweetened fruit juice.** (It is highly recommended to choose fruit over juice.)

Examples: Apple or orange, one small piece

## Non-Starchy Vegetables

**One serving equals 25 calories.**

**One serving equals half cup cooked vegetables or one cup raw vegetables.**

Some Examples:

- Asparagus
- Green Beans
- Beets
- Broccoli
- Carrots
- Cooking Greens (collard, kale, mustard, turnip, spinach)
- Salad Greens (endive, lettuce, romaine), also on free list
- Squash (summer)
- Tomatoes
- Zucchini

## Starch

**Each serving equals 80 calories.**

### Cereals/grains/pasta
Cooked cereals, half cup
Ready-to-eat unsweetened cereals, three quarters cup
Pasta (cooked); rice, white or brown (cooked), one third cup

### Starchy vegetables
Corn, peas, half cup
Potato, baked, one quarter large (3 oz.)
Winter squash, one cup

### Bread/crackers/snacks (generally, a serving is one ounce or 80 calories of a bread or starchy snack)
one ounce serving of bread, bagels, rolls (choose whole grain)
Organic Triscuits, four crackers

## Protein: Meat, Poultry, and Meat Substitutes (Limiting red meat is recommended)

### Lean options
**One serving equals one ounce and is 45 calories.**
One ounce fish or shellfish; one ounce poultry without the skin
Pork (lean cuts), one ounce
Lean beef (choose leaner cuts such as sirloin), one ounce
Light cheese, one ounce
Egg whites, two

### Medium/High-Fat Protein Selections
**Count the meat/cheese items in this category as one protein and one fat. Each item below equals 75 to 100 calories per ounce.**

Beef and pork (fattier cuts and ground) one ounce, (limit red meat)

Eggs, one

Bacon, three slices (limit red meat)

Regular Cheese (not light or fat free), one ounce

## Protein: Plant-Based Substitutes

Peanut butter, one tablespoon

Tofu, half cup

Beans, half cup (count as one protein plus half starch)

Veggie patty, count as two proteins plus half starch (for a patty that is around 130 calories)

## Milk

**One serving equals 100 calories**

Skim or 1% milk, one cup

Yogurt – look on label: every 100 calories of yogurt is one serving

Milk substitutes (soy milk, rice milk, almond milk – look for calcium-fortified brands. Look at label: 100 calories is one milk serving). Serving size can vary. A good estimate is roughly a cup.

## Fats

**Each serving equals 45 calories. In general, one teaspoon of an oil is one fat serving.**

**Unsaturated Fats**

Avocado, two tablespoons (one ounce)

Peanut butter, half tablespoon

Mayonnaise, 1 teaspoon

Nuts: almonds or cashews (six nuts), peanuts (10 nuts), pecans (four halves)

Seeds: sesame, pumpkin, sunflower, one tablespoon

Olives, eight to ten

Salad dressing with oil, one tablespoon

Oil, one teaspoon

**Saturated Fats (Limit)**

Bacon, one slice

Butter, one teaspoon

Cream cheese, regular one tablespoon

Cream, half and half, two tablespoons

## Please note that:

**One Carbohydrate serving equals one Starch or one Milk or one Fruit**

## Free Foods

Some have a small number of calories, so moderation is key.

**Drinks**

Bouillon or broth

Club soda, carbonated water, or mineral water

Coffee or tea

Soft drinks, diet, sugar-free (Limit, and then eventually cut out diet drinks, and drinks with sweeteners whether artificial or natural)

**Condiments/seasonings**

Fresh herbs

Flavoring extract (buy organic)

Garlic

Lemon juice

Pepper

Vinegar

**Vegetables (Free)**

Leafy Greens

# Thank You

Thank you so much for choosing to read this book. I appreciate your time investment! Now, I hope you invest in the strategies discussed so that you can enjoy infinite nutrition and wellness dividends!

Please share this book with others. Please share your feedback with me, and tell me how this book has helped you. Any suggestions or tips for future books are welcome. Please consider writing a review for my book, as word-of-mouth truly helps independent authors.

Let's stay connected. Follow me on these social media sites for nutrition tips, updates, and fun information.

**Facebook:** Facebook.com/Tricia.Silverman
**Instagram:** Instagram.com/TriciaSilverman/
**Twitter:** Twitter.com/TriciaSilverman
**LinkedIn:** https://bit.ly/2RqpeeG
Please check out my website at TriciaSilverman.com.
Contact me at http://www.triciasilverman.com/contact or tricia@triciasilverman.com

Please consider having me speak at your next event and refer me to any groups you know of that are looking for a dynamic nutrition presentation.

I look forward to staying in touch!

–Tricia

# WANT MORE OF TRICIA'S GUIDANCE?

- Hire Tricia as a speaker for your next conference, workplace event, spa, or senior center gathering.

- Hire Tricia as your fitness or nutrition coach.

Get on Tricia's mailing list for updates on nutrition news, new books, and services. Sign up at the bottom of Tricia's homepage at: **http://www.triciasilverman.com**

- Download the bonus chapter at TriciaSilverman.com/book

# Tricia Silverman

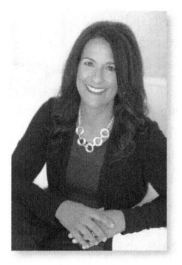

Tricia has been a fitness and nutrition enthusiast since she was a child. She graduated *summa cum laude* with a Bachelor of Science degree in dietetics from the State University of New York at Oneonta. She completed her dietetic internship at Brigham and Women's Hospital. She also graduated with honors from the Babson College MBA program.

She is a registered dietitian, certified wellness coach through Wellcoaches, and a fitness instructor (certified as a personal trainer through ACE and a group fitness instructor through AFAA). She has extensive nutrition education experience, including time spent as the director of nutrition for the prestigious Canyon Ranch Health Resort in the Berkshires.

During her employment with the Boston Public Schools, she taught nutrition and was responsible for the operations of over 20 school nutrition meal sites, which employed over 100 people. Her vast school nutrition and management experience also includes three years as the director of food services at Watertown Public Schools, where she was responsible for operations and developed and implemented innovative nutrition education opportunities for the students.

She owns Tricia Silverman Wellness, a nutrition and wellness consulting firm in Massachusetts. She has been in business since 2004. Her company specializes in high energy, fun, and informative wellness programs, including combined nutrition and fitness programs, innovative nutrition presentations, health fair services, business consulting, article writing, and customized individual nutrition/wellness coaching sessions. She is an international professional speaker and speaks at employee sites, senior centers, businesses, conferences, and more!

She created and leads the Active Aging Nutrition Certification for SCW Fitness Education Company and won the title of Fitness Presenter of the Year for SCW's 2018 Florida fitness convention. She also won the title of SCW Fitness Mania Boston Fitness Idol Competition in 2016. She has spoken across the US at over 20 SCW Fitness Education Company conferences since 2017. She has spoken at two canfitpro Toronto conferences. In 2019, she presented at the International Council on Active Aging Conference in Florida. Since 2011, she has been speaking annually at the Massachusetts Councils on Aging state conferences.

The Dietitian's in Business and Communications practice group honored her with the Circle Award in 2006 for her outstanding contribution to the group as newsletter editor. She was named the 2008 Chapter Member of the Year by the National Speakers Association New England, and the 2008 Recognized Young Dietitian of the Year Award by the Massachusetts Dietetic Association. She was the state liaison for the Nutrition Entrepreneurs Dietetic Practice Group in Massachusetts from 2004 to 2015. She served on the board of directors for the National Speakers Association New England Chapter for two years. Tricia has been published in *Bipolar Magazine* and *Schizophrenia Digest,* as well as other mental health magazines. She has been quoted in blogs and numerous articles. She has written articles for the canfitpro magazine and blog, and SCW's Spotlight publication. Tricia has been teaching Nutrition Entrepreneurship for the Master's in Applied Nutrition Program at Northeastern University for 12 years! Tricia also has taught Nutrition Entrepreneurship for the University of Saint Joseph. Additionally, she teaches Healthy Aging: Nutrition Strategies for Optimal Longevity for Northeastern University.

**Her website is TriciaSilverman.com, and she can be reached at Tricia@TriciaSilverman.com.**

# Endnotes

1   The Staff of Canyon Ranch, Sherman L. The Canyon Ranch Guide to Living Younger Longer. Simon and Schuster; 2001.

2   Banik A, Taylor R. Hunza Land, The Fabulous Health and Youth Wonderland of the World. Whitehorn Publishing; 1960.

3   Wang D, Li Y, Chiuve S, Stampfer M, et al. Association of specific dietary fats with total and cause-specific mortality. *JAMA Intern Med.* 2016;176(8):1134–1145.

4   Chernoff C. Carbohydrate, Fat, and Fluid Requirements in: Older Adults. *Geriatric Nutrition The Health Professional's Handbook.* 4th ed. Burlington, MA: Jones & Bartlett Learning; 2014:27-31.

5   Bernstein M, Plawecki K. Macronutrient and Fluid Recommendations and Alcohol in Older Adults. In: Bernstein M, Munoz N. *Nutrition For Older Adults.* Burlington, MA: Jones & Bartlett Learning; 2016:62-66.

6   Somer E. Food & Mood: *The Complete Guide to Eating Well and Feeling Your Best.* 2nd ed. New York, NY: Henry Holt and Company, LLC; 1999.

7   Schnabel L, Kesse-Guyot E, Allès B, et al. Association between ultraprocessed food consumption and risk of mortality among middle-aged adults in France. *JAMA Intern Med.* 2019;179(4):490–498. https://jamanetwork.com/journals/jamainternalmedicine/article-abstract/2723626.

8   Ibid.

9   Food and Drug Administration Website. Overview of Food Ingredients, Additives & Colors. https://www.fda.gov/food/ingredientspackaginglabeling/foodadditivesingredients/ucm094211.htm. Accessed 8/19/18.

10  Food and Drug Administration Website. What We Do. https://www.fda.gov/aboutfda/whatwedo/default.htm. Accessed 8/29/18.

11  Singh R, Ishikawa S. Food additive P-80 impacts mouse gut microbiota promoting intestinal inflammation, obesity and liver dysfunction. *SOJ microbiology & infectious diseases.* 2016;4(1):10.

12  Lecithin Bleached. United States Department of Agriculture. Agricultural Marketing Service. 8/6/09. https://www.ams.usda.gov/sites/default/files/media/Lecithin%20bleached%20TR%202009.pdf. Accessed 9/5/18.

13  Q3C — Tables and List Guidance for Industry. Food and Drug Administration Website. June 2017. https://www.fda.gov/regulatory-information/search-fda-guidance-documents/q3c-tables-and-list-rev-3. Accessed 9/4/18.

14  Directive 2009/32/EC of the European Parliament and of the Council of 23 April 2009 on the approximation of the laws of the Member States on extraction solvents used in the production of foodstuffs and food ingredients (Recast) (Text with EEA relevance). https://eur-lex.europa.eu/legal-content/EN/TXT/?uri=CELEX:02009L0032-20100916. Accessed 9/4/18.

15  Markowitz T. All About Food: The manufacturing of our food is not pretty. LA Times. JAN 27, 2015. http://www.latimes.com/tn-hbi-et-0129-all-about-food-yucky-foods-20150127-story.html. Accessed 9/4/18.

16  Behind the Bean The Heroes and Charlatans of the Natural and Organic Soy Foods Industry. Cornucopia Institute. 2009. https://www.cornucopia.org/wp-content/uploads/2017/09/behindthebean_color_final.pdf. Accessed 9/4/18.

17  Food and Drug Administration Website. Letter posted July 7, 2017 from USDA to Cargill Representative. https://www.fda.gov/media/106779/download. Accessed 11/20/18.

18  USDA Website. Safety Health and Environmental Training. Hexanes. https://www.ars.usda.gov/northeast-area/docs/safety-health-and-environmental-training/hexanes/. Accessed 9/4/18.

19  Environmental Protection Agency. Toxicological Review of n-Hexane. https://cfpub.epa.gov/ncea/iris/iris_documents/documents/toxreviews/0486tr.pdf. November 2005. Accessed 9/18/2018.

20  Rodriguez-Palacios A, et al. The artificial sweetener splenda promotes gut proteobacteria, dysbiosis, and myeloperoxidase reactivity in Crohn's disease–like ileitis, *Inflammatory Bowel Diseases*, 2008;24(5):1005-1020. https://academic.oup.com/ibdjournal/article/24/5/1005/4939054. Accessed 1/19/19.

21  Ibid.

22  Hamishehkar H, Khani S, Kashanian S, Ezzati Nazhad Dolatabadi J, Eskandani M. Geno- and cytotoxicity of propyl gallate food additive. *Drug & Chemical Toxicology* [serial online]. July 2014;37(3):241-246. Available from: Academic Search Complete, Ipswich, MA. Accessed 9/9/18.

23  Speijers G, van Apeldoorn M. Gallates (Propyl, Octyl And Dodecyl). IPCS: International Program on Chemical Safety. http://www.inchem.org/documents/jecfa/jecmono/v32je02.htm National Institute of Public Health and Environmental Protection, Laboratory for Toxicology, Bilthoven, The Netherlands. Accessed 9/10/18.

24  Gray J, Rasanayagam S, Engel C, Rizzo J. State of the evidence 2017: an update on the connection between breast cancer and the environment. *Environmental Health*. 2017;16:94. https://www.ncbi.nlm.nih.gov/pubmed/28865460. Accessed on June 27, 2019.

25  Winters R. *Consumer's Dictionary of Food Additives*. Fifth Edition. New York, NY: Three Rivers Press; 1999.

26  McDonald C. Food Dive. May 18, 2018. https://www.fooddive.com/news/health-advocates-sue-fda-for-failure-to-ban-7-artificial-flavors/523287/. Accessed 9/15/18.

27  Center for Science in the Public interest. Chemical Cuisine. Center for Science in the Public Interest Website https://cspinet.org/eating-healthy/chemical-cuisine#artificialcolorings. Accessed 9/14/18.

28  Ritz E, Hahn K, Ketteler M, Kuhlmann MK, Mann J. Phosphate additives in food—a health risk. *Dtsch Arztebl Int*. 2012;109(4):49–55. https://www.ncbi. nlm.nih.gov/pubmed/22334826. Accessed 6/1/19.

29  Ibid.

30  World Health Organization. Foods, Genetically Modified. World Health Organization website. http://www.who.int/topics/food_genetically_modified/en/. Accessed 9/10/18.

31  Non-GMO Project. GMO Facts. The Non-GMO Project Website. https://www.nongmoproject.org/gmo-facts/. Accessed 12/30/18.

32  Bøhn T, Cuhra M, Traavik T, Sanden M, Fagan J, Primicerio R. Compositional differences in soybeans on the market: glyphosate accumulates in Roundup Ready GM soybeans. *Food Chem*. 2013. https://www.ncbi.nlm.nih.gov/pubmed/24491722. Accessed 12/30/18.

33  "FDA In Brief: Final results from FDA's Pesticide Monitoring Report shows pesticide residues in foods below federal limits." US Food and Drug Administration. October 1, 2018. https://www.fda.gov/news-events/fda-brief/ fda-brief-final-results-fdas-pesticide-monitoring-report-shows-pesticide- residues-foods-below. Accessed 5-17-19.

34  USDA Organic Labeling Standards. United States Department of Agriculture. https://www.ams.usda.gov/grades-standards/organic-labeling-standards. Accessed 9/11/18.

35  United State Department of Agriculture. Understanding the Price Tag. Choose My Plate website. https://www.choosemyplate.gov/budget-price-tag. Accessed 9/11/18. The noted website is no longer offering the link to unit pricing.

36  Pase, M, Himali, J, et al. Sugary beverage intake and preclinical Alzheimer's disease in the community. *Alzheimer's and Dementia*. 2017; 13 (9): 955-964.

37  Tey S, Salleh N, Henry J, Forde C. Effects of aspartame-, monk fruit-, stevia- and sucrose-sweetened beverages on postprandial glucose, insulin and energy intake. *Int J Obes*, 2017: Mar;41(3):450-457. https://www.ncbi.nlm.nih.gov/ pubmed/27956737. Epub 2016 Dec 13. Accessed 5/20/19.

38  Muñoz-García M, et al. (2019) Sugar-sweetened and artificially-sweetened beverages and changes in cognitive function in the SUN project, *Nutritional Neuroscience*, https://www.ncbi.nlm.nih.gov/pubmed/30794108. Accessed 5/20/19.

39  Gardener H, Rundek T, Markert M, Wright CB, Elkind MS, Sacco RL. Diet soft drink consumption is associated with an increased risk of vascular events in the Northern Manhattan Study. *J Gen Intern Med*. 2012;27(9):1120-1126. https://www.ncbi.nlm.nih.gov/pmc/articles/PMC3514985/. Accessed 5-19-19.

40  Nall R. Does the 20-20-20 rule prevent eye stain? Medical News Today website. 4-18-18. Accessed on 5-19-19.

41  Aspinall P, Mavros P, Coyne R, et al. The urban brain: analysing outdoor physical activity with mobile EEG. *British Journal of Sports Medicine.* 2015;49:272-276.

42  U.S. Department of Health and Human Services. Physical Activity Guidelines for Americans 2nd edition. Office of Disease Prevention and Health Promotion Website. https://health.gov/paguidelines/second-edition/pdf/Physical_Activity_Guidelines_2nd_edition.pdf. 2018. Accessed 5/1/19.

43  Ibid.

44  Fletcher H. The A.B.- Z. of Our Own Nutrition. New York: Frederick A. Stokes Company; 1903.

45  Tuoyire DA. Television exposure and overweight/obesity among women in Ghana. *BMC obesity.* 2018;5:8. https://www.ncbi.nlm.nih.gov/pubmed/29468075.

46  Halliday J. Thin Within: A grace-oriented Approach to Lasting Weight Loss. 2nd edition. Nashville, TN: Thomas Nelson Publishers; 2005.

47  Garaulet M, Gómez-Abellán P, Alburquerque-Béjar J, Lee Y, Ordovás J, Scheer F. Timing of food intake predicts weight loss effectiveness. *Int J Obes (Lond).* 2013;37(4):604-11.

48  Flood-Obbagy J, Rolls B. "The effect of fruit in different forms on energy intake and satiety at a meal." *Appetite.* 2009 Apr;52(2):416-22. https://www.ncbi.nlm.nih.gov/pmc/articles/PMC2664987/. Accessed 1/2/19.

49  Raines, et al. Hoarding and eating pathology: The mediating role of emotion regulation. *Comprehensive Psychiatry.* 2015;57(C):29–35.

50  Parry D, Oeppen R, Gass H, Brennan P. Impact of hydration and nutrition on personal performance in the clinical workplace. *British Journal of Oral & Maxillofacial Surgery.* December 2017;55(10):995-998.

51  Conner T, Brookie K, Richardson A, Polak M. On carrots and curiosity: Eating fruit and vegetables is associated with greater flourishing in daily life. *Br J Health Psychol.* 2015;20:413-427. https://onlinelibrary.wiley.com/doi/abs/10.1111/bjhp.12113. Accessed 1/2/19.

52  Anastasiou C, Yannakoulia M, Kosmidis M, et al. Mediterranean diet and cognitive health: Initial results from the Hellenic Longitudinal Investigation of Ageing and Diet. *PLoS ONE.* 2017; 12(8)9.

53  Breus M. *The Sleep Doctor's Diet Plan*; New York, NY: Rodale; 2011.

54  Batista C and Almeida L. Disease and Conditions in the Older Adults Nutritional Implications- Cognitive Disorders. In: Bernstein M, Munoz N. *Nutrition for the Older Adult.* Burlington, MA: Jones and Bartlett Learning: 2016: 289-304.

55  Agrawal R, Gomez -Pinilla G. 'Metabolic syndrome' in the brain: deficiency in omega-3 fatty acid exacerbates dysfunctions in insulin receptor signaling and cognition. *Journal of Physiology.* 2012;590.10:2485-2499.

56  Academy of Nutrition and Dietetics: Food and Nutrition for Older Adults: Promoting Health and Wellness. *Journal of the Academy of Nutrition and Dietetics.* 2012;112(8):1255–1277.

57  Crichton, G, Bryan J, Murphy K. Dietary Antioxidants, Cognitive Function and Dementia - A Systematic Review. *Plant Foods Hum Nutr.* 2013;68:279.

58  Ibid.

59  Liu, RH. Health benefits of fruit and vegetables are from additive and synergistic combinations of phytochemicals. *The Journal of Nutrition Health and Aging.* 2012;16,(7).

60  Ibid.

61  Loef M, Walach H. Fruit, vegetables and prevention of cognitive decline or dementia: A systematic review of cohort studies. *J Nutr Health Aging.* 2012; 16:626.

62  Ibid.

63  Batista C, Almeida L. Disease and Conditions in the Older Adults Nutritional Implications-Cognitive Disorders. In: Bernstein M, Munoz N. *Nutrition for the Older Adult.* Burlington, MA: Jones and Bartlett Learning: 2016.

64  Roberts R, Geda Y, Cerhan J, et al. Vegetables, unsaturated fats, moderate alcohol intake, and mild cognitive impairment. *Dementia and Geriatric Cognitive Disorders.* 2010;29(5):413-423.

65  Batista C, Almeida L. Disease and Conditions in the Older Adults Nutritional Implications-Cognitive Disorders. In: Bernstein M, Munoz N. *Nutrition for the Older Adult.* Burlington, MA: Jones and Bartlett Learning: 2016.

66  Ibid.

67  Ibid.

68  Ibid.

69  Panza F, Solfrizzi V, Logroscino G, et al. Coffee, tea, and caffeine consumption and prevention of late-life cognitive decline and dementia: A systematic review. *Journal of Nutrition, Health & Aging* [serial online]. March 2015;19(3):313-328. Available from: CINAHL Complete, Ipswich, MA. Accessed 2/24/18.

70  U.S. Department of Health and Human Services and U. S. Department of Agriculture. *2015-2020 Dietary Guidelines for Americans.* 8th Edition. 2015. https://health.gov/dietaryguidelines/2015/.

71  Ibid.

72  Pase MP, Himali JJ, Beiser AS, et al. Sugar- and artificially sweetened beverages and the risks of incident stroke and dementia. *Stroke.* 2017;48:1139-1146.

73  National Sleep Foundation. Understanding Sleep Cycles: What Happens While You Sleep. Sleep.org website. https://www.sleep.org/articles/what-happens-during-sleep/. Accessed 1/3/19.

74  Wurtman J, Frusztajer N. *The Serotonin Power Diet.* New York, NY: Rodale; 2006.

75  Arpaia J, Rapgay L. *Real Meditation in Minutes a Day.* Somerville, MA. Wisdom Publications; 2008.

76   Ross A, Brooks A, Touchton-Leonard K, et al. A different weight loss experience: A qualitative study exploring the behavioral, physical, and psychosocial changes associated with yoga that promote weight loss. *Evidence-Based Complementary and Alternative Medicine.* 2016.

77   Worthington E. Reach Forgiveness of Others. Everett Worthington website. http://www.evworthington-forgiveness.com/reach-forgiveness-of-others. Accessed 1-13-19.

78   Neff K. What is Self-Compassion? Self-Compassion-org website. https://self-compassion.org/#. Accessed 1-13-19.

79   Prochaska, J, DiClemente C. *The transtheoretical approach: Crossing the traditional boundaries of therapy.* Melbourne, Florida: Krieger Publishing Company 1984.

80   Make a Vision Board. What is a Vision Board. Makeavisionboard.com website. https://www.makeavisionboard.com/what-is-a-vision-board/. Accessed 1/13/19.

81   Morin A. How a Sense of Purpose Adds Years to Your Life, According to Scientists. Inc.com. https://www.inc.com/amy-morin/science-explains-how-a-sense-of-purpose-adds-years-to-your-life.html. April 14, 2016. Accessed 2/15/19.

82   Willcox B, Wilcox C, Suzuki M. *The Okinawa Program.* Three Rivers Press; 2001.

83   Buettner D. *The Blue Zones Solution, Eating and Living Like the World's Healthiest People.* National Geographic; 2015.

84   Robbins J. *Healthy at 100.* Ballantine Books; 2007.

85   Young P. 161 Years Old and Going Strong. *Life Magazine.* Volume 65 Issue 12. September 16, 1966.

86   Young R, Desjardins B, McLaughlin K, Poulain M, Perls T. Typologies of Extreme Longevity Myths. *Current Gerontology and Geriatrics Research.* 2010;2010:423087. https://www.hindawi.com/journals/cggr/2010/423087/. Accessed 1/19/19.

87   Ibid.

88   Robbins J. *Healthy at 100.* Ballantine Books; 2007.

89   Buettner D. *The Blue Zones: Nine Lessons for Living Longer from the People Who've Lived the Longest.* National Geographic; 2012.

90   Robbins J. *Healthy at 100.* Ballantine Books; 2007.

91   Miller M, Mente A, Dehghan M, et al. Fruit, vegetable, and legume intake, and cardiovascular disease and deaths in 18 countries (PURE): a prospective cohort study. *The Lancet.* 2017;390(10107)2037-2049.

92   Robbins J. *Healthy at 100.* Ballantine Books; 2007.

93   Rodale J. *The Healthy Hunzas.* Rodale Press; 1948.

94   Banik A, Taylor R. Hunza Land, The Fabulous Health and Youth Wonderland of the World. Whitehorn Publishing; 1960.

95   Ibid.

96    Ibid.

97    Ibid.

98    Buettner D. The Blue Zones Solution, Eating and Living Like the World's
      Healthiest People National Geographic; 2015.

99    Willcox B, Wilcox C, Suzuki M. *The Okinawa Program*. Three Rivers Press; 2001.

100   Trichopoulou A, Bamia, C, Trichopoulos D, Anatomy of health effects
      of Mediterranean diet: Greek EPIC prospective cohort study. *BMJ*
      2009;338:b2337 http://www.bmj.com/content/338/bmj.b2337. Accessed on
      6/19/19.

101   Anastasiou C et al. Mediterranean diet linked with improved cognitive
      performance in elderly. *PLOS One*. 2017 August 1. 12(8).

102   Ibid.

103   Choose Your Food Exchange Lists for Weight Management. American
      Diabetes Association Academy of Nutrition and Dietetics. 2008.